GIVEN UP ON EXERCISE?

YOUR FOOLPROOF PATH TO LASTING FITNESS

By Michele Silence M.A.

IngramSpark 2025

ISBN (Paperback): 978-0-9893133-1-5

Printed in the United States of America

DEDICATION

For all my students over the past 45 years—from my youngest preschoolers to the adults who have remained in my classes through the years. You have taught me as much as I have taught you and have proven that fitness is truly timeless.

PREFACE

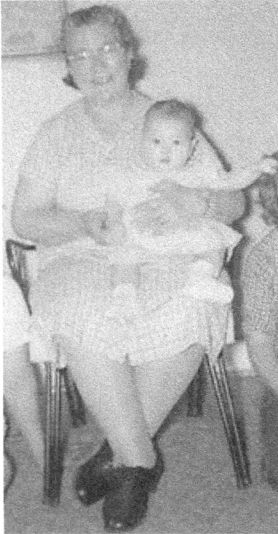

This is me and my grandmother. I get it. I grew up in an Italian/Polish family. Food was plentiful. And delicious. I was called "chubby" during the first 12 years of my life. Exercise? What was that? I do remember a few times my mom tried to get in some Jack LaLanne exercises while I watched intently. That didn't last long. Then there was the plastic sauna suit. I think she did that once. She tried eating those Ayds weight loss candies (basically an appetite suppressant loaded with sugar and caffeine). It resembled chewy chocolate so I was always sneaking into the box to eat them. Like the chocolate laxatives, but I only ate those once. Of course none of those things helped her to lose weight. We were all still eating bacon and eggs for breakfast, meatballs and cheesy lasagna for dinner and homemade calorie laden desserts every night.

No one in my family did any exercise. My dad worked long hours, my mom had to do almost everything in the household and take care of four of us kids. At home, I'd just sit and read or watch TV like everyone else. I learned how to do just about every sedentary activity. Make potholders out of looms, knit, crochet, sew, put together puzzles, and got good doing all kinds of crafts. Had it not been for my grandfather, I would never have even learned how to swing a bat, ride a bike or swim.

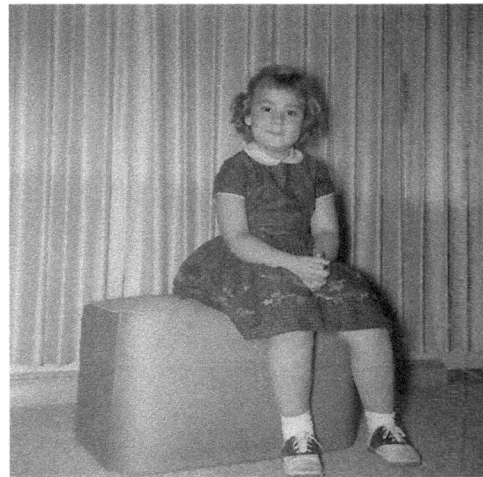

Needless to say I was an overweight and out of shape child. Picked on constantly. My brother called me "Fat and Ugly." I was so big I couldn't even get on a horse. My one attempt at a campground pony ride got the horse so upset he threw me off and stomped

iv

on my foot. My school classmates got a hold of my report card (weight was noted on it) and called me "Elephant Legs." I couldn't finish any of the classroom Presidential Fitness Tests. The 600-yard run may as well have been a 600 mile marathon to me. I always walked most of it, out of breath. Coming in last and ashamed, as if I was to blame instead of the teacher for not providing conditioning ahead of time. I wanted so much to be a cheerleader but never made the team. To make things worse, exercise was used for punishment. Come late to class? Do 50 push-ups. Be last on the run? Do 10 more laps. With those kinds of consequences, how could I possibly develop a love for physical activity? I despised anything that had to do with P.E. No wonder.

At the age of 21, I was trapped in a cycle of overeating, watching the numbers on the scale climb higher and higher. At that time I moved across the country to strike out on my own. It wasn't until I was 23 and going through a divorce that I was lucky enough to have a friend take me to an aerobics class. It was in the 1980's so there were lots of leg warmers, leotards, and fun, energizing music. I did one class and said to myself "I can do this!" Better yet, I liked it! That was the beginning of a whole new life for me. For the first time ever I was able to get in shape. I lost fat and gained muscle. It was fun going to class and the people I met were great, they made me laugh. Surprisingly, this became a habit. I felt good, I looked good, my self-esteem went up and mood improved. I was even ready to take on some painful psychological issues through therapy.

Eventually, I bought a fitness studio, learned to teach aerobics, got certified and held specialty classes that no one else was doing at the time. Aerobics classes for seniors. And aerobics classes for overweight students, called Largercise. Those classes took off and I saw how these two groups of people had nowhere to turn to when it came to appropriate exercise programs. Those classes continued for years. Not only did I get to see miraculous changes in the students, but I learned about their mindsets. The things that they were fearful of, the past traumas that kept them from focusing on their bodies, thoughts of inferiority and more. It was then I realized that getting and staying fit had more to do with the mind than the body. When people feel safe, they can open up, learn and achieve. At that point I went back to school and earned my master's degree in psychology.

When my son was born, I started doing counseling with adults but found myself pulled in a different direction. To help create fitness programming for young preschool children. They need to learn that exercise is fun from the start. Instilling how to make healthy food choices before they are too set with unhealthy habits. So, in addition to instructing my adult students, I was also running what became an international preschool fitness program called KID-FIT. Something that I enjoyed doing for the next 30 years.

Today I am a fitness consultant, personal trainer, writer, educator, and preschool fitness expert. None of this would have happened without changing my mental and physical health. I got clinical therapy—good therapy—and started exercising. Those two things changed my life. I went from deep depression to a fulfilling, healthy life. We all need both mental and physical health to enjoy life to the fullest.

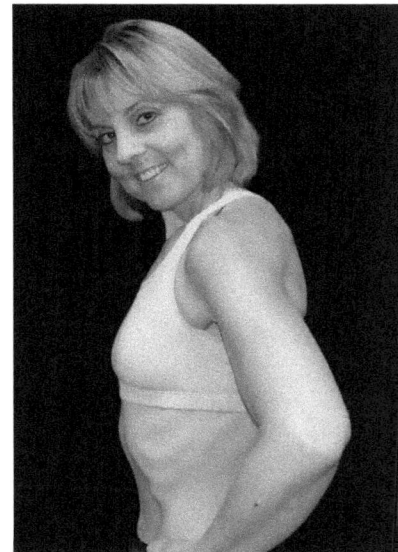

Whether you share some of the above experiences or have your own equally compelling stories, this book is for you. It doesn't matter how many times you've tried and quit. It doesn't matter how old you are. What matters is that you care about yourself and your health. That you want to get stronger and healthier from where you are today.

This workbook won't contain strict diets, impossible workouts or anything extreme. My approach is a sensible, day-by-day system. One that builds upon small steps. One thing at a time. Slowly, gradually and with lots of learning along the way. Learning not only about fitness but about you and why getting in shape may or may not have worked for you in the past. For the past 45 years I've helped people get and stay fit. I know the struggles. My goal for you is to help you get started in a safe, comfortable way with a program designed just for you. The goal being not just to start a program, but to continue an exercise program throughout your life. It can be done. The most difficult part is truly that first step. If you can take that first step, I'll be here to help you along the rest of your journey. That first step starts here, as soon as you turn the page.

TABLE OF CONTENTS

Part 1: Understanding Yourself to Set the Foundation

Focus on self-reflection, identifying psychological barriers, and setting the mental foundation for success.

Part 2: Building Knowledge and Learning the Basics

Learn the essential components of exercise, covering both science and practical skills.

Part 3: Creating and Committing to Your Personalized Plan

Design your individualized fitness program, commit to it, and track your progress.

Part 4: Practical Guidance

Advice on equipment, injury prevention, weight loss aids, and finding professional support.

Part 5: Progress, Reflection, and Sustainability

Maintain long-term success by reflecting on your journey and planning adaptations. Includes testimonials and space for your fitness diary, reflections, and stage-of-change revisits.

Appendices

INTRODUCTION

So you want to get fit? Is it really possible? Maybe you've started before and given up or simply lacked the motivation to keep going. Perhaps you've always hated the thought or simply didn't care. You know exercise is good for you and that you'd feel better if you did it, but just where do you start? It seems so complicated and daunting.

If you've asked yourself these questions, the fact that you're even reading these words shows there is hope for you. Somewhere, deep down inside, you really do yearn to be in better shape. Finding out how and having help each step of the way is finally at your fingertips.

There are many reasons why people find it difficult to start and stick with a fitness program. Probably the biggest one is that they didn't learn physical skills and develop a love of movement from a young age. Imagine if you were never taught to wash your hands, comb your hair, or take a bath. What if you had to make a conscious decision to do those things every single day? Fortunately, we don't. We were taught those things so early on that we automatically do them. When was the last time you thought about brushing your teeth? Wondering if you should or shouldn't? No, instead you automatically do it. It's a habit, learned from day one. It goes back so far you probably don't even remember the first time you brushed. Imagine if exercise was like that. Unfortunately for many people, it's not. That's not your fault.

Exercise is often viewed negatively in our society. Where are the incentives ($$) from insurance companies to help people get and stay healthy? Newscasters make jokes about how unfit they are. Fitness boot camps advertise they'll push your limits to get you into shape. Scammers are always out there promising a new potion to help you lose weight without moving a muscle. Is it any wonder why it's so easy to throw your arms up in the air and say, "What's the use?"

Over time we have gradually let our children down. Families aren't as active as they used to be. It's great that we don't have to work in fields anymore, but many of us sit at desks or do mundane jobs that tax more of our minds than our bodies. In fact, most of us are so overworked that the last thing we want to do when we come home is something physical. TV, mobile devices and computers have been overly welcomed into the home to babysit children and take the place of family interaction and activity. But even more importantly, we've denied our kids the opportunity to learn the skills necessary to maintain and enjoy physical fitness throughout life. Learning to move and enjoy exercise starts at birth.

It's not just the family that's responsible either. When funds get scarce, physical education programs get cut from public schools. In all but a few states, youth no longer have daily opportunities to learn basic skills in school such as kicking, throwing, catching, striking, and jumping. They have no structured PE programs. When those kids reach their teenage years, unless they're natural-born athletes, they'll feel too unequipped to participate in sports. Is there a teenager out there who wants to be embarrassed by not being able to hit the tennis or volleyball? So, kids shy away from sports and other forms of physical activity and opt for more sedentary activities. Then, once we reach adulthood those feelings of inadequacy can be strong. They can easily and unconsciously steer one away from movement.

If you are a non-exerciser, you have plenty of company. In the United States, the Centers for Disease Control and Prevention (CDC) reports that only 24% of adults get enough exercise to do themselves any good. That's not very many - and the reason for skyrocketing levels of heart disease, stroke, diabetes, and a slew of other diseases of lifestyle.

It's also not your fault that the fitness industry was never designed to actually help those who are deconditioned or overweight. Clubs make money on how many memberships they sell, not on how many people use the facility or get results. It's hard to learn what to do, when, how often, and how to do so safely. Where do you even start? No one wants to feel self-conscious walking into a gym for the first time. So for many, the first time is also the last.

The world moves fast. Family takes up a lot of time. So does work. It's easy to get overwhelmed and feel like there just isn't time or that you're too tired. Maybe you're older or have a physical condition and you're afraid you won't be able to do much. What about money? Whose got funds for equipment, memberships, or fitness classes? You can't imagine exercise being enjoyable anyway – you have no positive frame of reference.

When you started to learn to use a computer, you didn't just plop down in front of the screen and start punching aimlessly away at the keyboard. Most likely you started by educating yourself about computers — what they are, how they work and which one to get. You learned which programs are best for what you want to do and how to run them. Obviously, all that learning couldn't have taken place in one day. This example seems so obvious, yet millions of people don't realize the same logic applies to exercise. Those eager to start exercising too often make the mistake of just "jumping into it." They try to get going on a program they genuinely want to work, but without enough of the basics. The result, of course, is not a healthier body. The result is more likely frustration, anger, depression, or trashing the whole idea.

That's why this book is in your hands. It will help you every step of the way on your journey to better health. Everything in it has been used with my clients over the past 45 years. Worksheets, calendars, plans, charts – all designed to help you learn about exercise, what you can expect, about myths vs. facts, and how to make your program work. You'll learn what movements pose a lower or higher risk of injury for you, how to design your very own tailor-made workout, and how to make fitness last a lifetime. Most of all, you'll learn about yourself. Why you feel the way you do, what the specific obstacles are in your way, and how to move past them.

Yes, you'll learn all these things, but—just like when you began to use a computer—you'll learn them one step at a time. This book is divided into short chapters, each brief enough to be read in a single sitting. For the very best results, read only one chapter at a time. Give yourself at least a day to let the information really sink in. Allow yourself to think about the information during the day, applying it to the rest of your life when possible. If there is a worksheet at the end of the chapter, complete it before moving on. Each chapter builds upon information given earlier — a progressive approach to understanding yourself in order to get fit.

I can't stress enough how important it is to read only one chapter at a time. The human brain learns best when fed short amounts of information at a time. Long hours packed with thought provoking concepts and new ideas don't sink in. Do you really want to take the time to read if you're not going to retain a great deal of the material? There's a lot to think about before getting started. A lot to learn about yourself. When you take the time to read and complete each chapter, and thoroughly understand the ideas before moving ahead, you'll learn absolutely everything you need to know about how to get started on an exercise program and how to make it REALLY work for you. Not just for a few weeks or months, but for a lifetime.

At the end of each chapter you'll find a reflection page. Complete it after you have read the chapter and done any worksheets, quizzes or plans. This will help you summarize what you have learned and assure you have processed the information in a way that is meaningful to you. By taking it one chapter at a time and really thinking about what you're learning, you'll be able to turn these lessons into habits that stick over time.

And just to put you at ease, if the only thing you change by the time you get to the end of this workbook is that you move more each day and have just a few healthier eating habits you did it! You made a change that will drastically improve your health and wellbeing. When you understand the basics, learn about yourself, and have the right tools, it really is that simple.

UNDERSTANDING YOUR FITNESS JOURNEY

Making lasting changes in your fitness habits doesn't happen all at once. Just like learning any new skill, building a sustainable exercise routine takes time, effort, and patience. The Transtheoretical Model of Change, also called the Stages of Change, is a simple way to understand the journey you go through when creating a new habit.

Everyone starts at a different place, and that's okay. Some people aren't even thinking about exercising yet, while others may be actively trying to create a routine. By identifying where you are right now, you can set realistic goals and understand that slipping back or facing obstacles is part of the process—not a failure. The model also shows that change is cyclical, not a straight line. You might move forward, pause, or even return to an earlier stage before making lasting progress.

As you read this book, consider which stage you are currently in. You'll return to this model after completing the book to see how far you've come and how your habits have shifted. Recognizing your current stage and following the steps from there will help you make meaningful, long-term changes—one chapter, one step, and one habit at a time.

THE STAGES OF CHANGE

The flowchart visually represents the Transtheoretical Model. Think of it as a roadmap for your fitness journey:

1. Precontemplation – You're not yet considering exercise or don't feel it's relevant.

2. Contemplation – You're thinking about becoming more active but haven't made a plan yet.

3. Preparation – You're making small steps toward change, like gathering information or trying short workouts.

4. Action – You've begun a regular exercise routine, consistently practicing new habits.

5. Maintenance – You've sustained your routine for several months and are focused on keeping it going.

6. Relapse – Sometimes setbacks happen. You might return to an earlier stage, which is normal, and the cycle continues.

The arrows in the flowchart below show that change isn't always linear. You may revisit stages or move forward and backward at different times. This is completely normal—progress often comes in cycles, not in one straight line.

How to use this flowchart:

- Identify your current stage.

- Revisit it after finishing the book to see how far you've progressed.

- Reflect on what helped you move forward and what barriers you overcame.

By reviewing this model, you'll see that lasting change is a step-by-step process, integrating each lesson from the book into your daily life, one habit at a time.

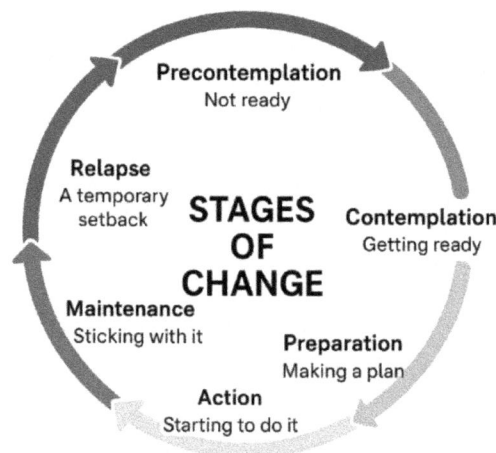

CHAPTER REFLECTION

Date: _____

What did I learn from this chapter?

What will I do differently or apply this week?

How do I feel after completing this chapter?

IT'S JUST A WORD

Exercise. It's just a word. Truly. In actuality exercise is described as physical activity that enhances or maintains fitness and overall health. That's a broad description. You already move all day long; how much more do you need to do in order for activity to count as exercise? Not a whole lot. And that is probably the biggest misconception held by people. It takes very little to improve your health and wellbeing.

But back to the word "exercise". What does it mean to you? If you grew up moving, doing sports, dancing, taking classes with friends, and going to the gym you would probably have a very different emotional response to the word than if you had always felt inadequate, laughed at, or felt physical pain. I know that firsthand. It takes a lot to change our emotional reactions to certain words but it can be done. The first thing is to understand how our emotions determine the power a simple word can have.

Any word can produce a negative or fearful reaction just as any word can be neutral or positive. It's all about our experiences, our personality and how we see the world. Particularly the past.

Below are some examples of different words. Think about how each word makes you feel. Note your initial reaction. Is it positive? Negative? Neutral? Words do not have power unless we assign power to them.

Complete the following task by looking at each word and recording what your initial emotional reaction to it is. Why do you have that reaction? Do you know why? If you do, is that reason still applicable? If not, why are you holding on to it?

WORD	REACTION (Good, Bad, Neutral)	WHY
Cup		
Dog		
Pillow		
Car		
Sing		
Exercise		
Doctor		
Daisy		
Bed		
Chocolate		

After doing the above activity, what have you learned about yourself? Do you have any insight now as to why it's been hard for you to start and stick with a fitness program? What trauma or experiences have you had that influenced your emotional response to the above words? Can you think of other words that trigger a negative emotional response that are affecting your life today?

So can you really reprogram your thinking? Absolutely! Instead of calling your program exercise, call it movement. Especially if you have no strong reaction to the word movement. Or start pairing the word 'exercise' with other things that are more pleasant so that it loses its negative charge.

Examples are relaxation exercise, breathing exercise or stretching exercise. Affirmations also work. Instead of thinking "I hate exercise", tell yourself "exercise is a way I take care of myself." The best way though is to replace those negative feelings with positive ones. You can do that by starting out with something so simple and so easy that it's non-threatening and fun. Make it doable and enjoyable.

Pick one of the above strategies that you feel would work best for you in changing what the word "exercise" means to you. Write it here and start using it:

_____

From this point on, start training your brain so that the word exercise does not hold a powerful grip over you. It's just a word. You don't need to fear it anymore. No one is going to hurt you, force you, ridicule you or make you do anything that you don't want to do for yourself. Not anymore.

CHAPTER REFLECTION

Date: _____

What did I learn from this chapter?

What will I do differently or apply this week?

How do I feel after completing this chapter?

SUCCESS, FAILURE AND MINDSET

Let's take a moment to reflect on what "success" and "failure" mean to you in the context of getting fit.

For you, does success mean exercising daily, achieving remarkable results, or even feeling ten years younger? Does it involve shedding excess weight and gaining the ability to tackle any physical challenge?

On the flip side, how do you define failure? If you set three fitness goals but only achieved one, would you see that as a failure? If you didn't meet any of your goals, would that feel like a total loss? Or could there be valuable lessons or positives to extract from your journey, regardless of the outcome?

Be careful of all-or-nothing thinking. If you have a habit of frequently using words like always, never, everyone, no one, all, none, completely, totally, must, impossible, forever, best and worst, those are very rigid. There's no middle ground.

These words leave no room for exceptions or uncertainty. Once you develop balanced thinking, you can accept outcomes that aren't black and white. You can view things on a spectrum rather than in extremes. You understand that more than one thing can be true at the same time. Like being able to enjoy a favorite snack and still be committed to eating healthy.

You can see that partial progress is still valuable. Balanced thinking encourages you to see in-between options and the potential for growth.

Lasting change doesn't come quick. Studies find that it typically takes around 66 days on average to form a new habit. New habit formation can range from 18 to 254 days, depending on the complexity of the behavior and the individual's consistency.

Numerous other studies suggest that complex behaviors (like exercising regularly) often take longer, sometimes taking between 100-254 days.

What does this tell you? It is pretty much impossible to break one habit (not exercising) and develop another one (regularly exercising) in a few weeks. Remind yourself it can take around 2 months or more for a new behavior to become a habit. Some habits form faster, some slower, depending on how complex they are and how consistently you practice. The key is small, repeated actions every day—not perfection. One thing at a time.

For a cigarette smoker, it takes 6 to 11 attempts to quit smoking before they succeed. Some studies suggest that it can even take up to 30 attempts for certain individuals, depending on various factors such as nicotine dependence, access to support, and personal motivation. Making dietary and physical activity changes is also an evolutionary process. It takes time. If you don't reach your goals the first attempt, keep trying! Each try brings you closer to your sustainable fitness routine and teaches you more about yourself.

A big part of it comes down whether your thought process is that of a "can do" or "can't do'" attitude. We refer to "can do" thinking as empowered thinking. This type of person has the ability to improve through effort, learning, and persistence, seeing challenges as opportunities for growth. The "can't do" attitude refers to limiting thinking. In other words, more apt to see abilities as static, viewing challenges as insurmountable and failure as a reflection of innate limitations. You've seen these mindsets in people you know and interact with every day. I find a lot of customer service reps are often "can't do" people. Whatever the issue may be, and whatever solution you propose, their answer is always, "We can't do that." Contrast that to the "can do" person. This person looks at things differently. If you ask for something, their first response is either yes or let's see how we "can do" that. They empathize with you and project the feeling they understand. Even if their answer works out to be the same as the "can't do" person, you feel better about it. You feel like someone actually listened to you, understood and validated your concern. Who wouldn't want that?

This is really important because this is how your brain tells you to react, automatically. This applies across various circumstances. Are you a "can do" or "can't do" type of person? Why do you think that is? Did you learn it? From whom? Is it comfortable? Why?

Look inside yourself to see which way your brain tends to gravitate. Try to understand why. And if it's not helping you get what you want in life, how can you change it?

WHY EXERCISE?

Next, examine why you actually want to exercise. By understanding why you want to exercise, you can develop a positive mindset that helps you approach the process in a healthy way. This mindset influences whether you view challenges as chances to improve or as reasons to quit. Knowing your motivations also helps you define success and failure, which is important for staying committed to exercise over time. What is it that keeps bringing you back to the starting block? Be clear on why you want to get and stay fit, whatever the reason(s). Jot them down and see if those reasons are the true reasons as you move through this workbook.

Reasons why I want to get and stay fit:

_____

_____

You might not be completely sure, and that's okay for now. However, you will become more highly focused on your "why" as we move ahead. As a motivational tool, consider the verified direct benefits of regular exercise that follow. *I've excluded weight loss to show that even if you never lose a pound, you can still enjoy these health benefits!*

Many times people start exercise programs for other reasons that are more important to them than weight loss so losing weight becomes an added benefit. Regular exercise not only helps to control weight but also allows you to enjoy all these benefits too. And that's not all. Check out the additional indirect benefits that come from a stable fitness routine on the last page.

Once you're on a sustainable, regular program you will gradually notice these benefits come to life. It might be at a doctor's appointment where you find out you don't have high blood pressure anymore. Or when you don't get tired walking around amusement parks any longer. Maybe you'll just find that you're in a better mood most of the time. Take a look at all the benefits there are to being fit. These things can stay with you for years if not forever. Read through the list and circle any that are especially important to you.

Verified Direct Benefits of Regular Exercise

(Circle those that are of particular importance to you)

Improves cardiovascular health	Improves digestion
Enhances mood	Reduces blood pressure
Boosts energy levels	Improves cholesterol levels
Strengthens muscles	Enhances insulin sensitivity
Increases bone density	Strengthens the core
Enhances brain function	Improves posture
Promotes better sleep	Increases lung capacity
Increases flexibility	Enhances athletic performance
Improves mobility	Promotes healthy aging
Enhances immune system	Improves circulation
Reduces chronic disease risk	Reduces risk of falls
Improves balance	Increases mental resilience
Enhances coordination	Reduces fatigue
Lowers stress	Improves joint health
Improves relaxation	Enhances self-esteem
Reduces inflammation	Reduces anxiety
Increases endurance	Improves social interaction
Enhances metabolism	Boosts cognitive function

Indirect Benefits of Regular Exercise

(Circle those that are of particular importance to you)

Enhanced Creativity

Enhanced Problem-Solving Skills

Increased Motivation

Improved Academic Performance

Greater Work Productivity

Better Coping Skills

Improved Quality of Life

Enhanced Longevity

Better Family Relationships

Increased Sense of Achievement

Improved Financial Well-Being

Improved Work-Life Balance

CHAPTER REFLECTION

Date: _____

What did I learn from this chapter?

What will I do differently or apply this week?

How do I feel after completing this chapter?

CONFRONTING FEARS, DITCHING EXCUSES

There's a saying, "Where the mind goes, the body will follow." It's true. If you're regularly telling yourself you're going to fail, most likely you will. If you have one negative thought after another, it's hard to stay motivated. Being positive is one of the top characteristics seen in people who live to be 100. So how can you reprogram yourself into being a more positive thinking person?

The first step is to be aware of how many times a day you think or say something negative. Print up a monthly calendar (a sample one is included at the end of this chapter). Every single time you have a negative thought or say something negative, make a mark on the day. See how long it will take before you preempt the negative comments and replace them with something else. For example, you may think, "I really don't feel like doing anything today." Instead, you can say "I know I'll feel better afterwards, even though I don't want to move."

It takes time to reprogram thoughts that you've had for a lifetime. Thoughts that once helped you survive trauma a long time ago may not be needed anymore. They cause stress and affect your health negatively. Being aware of the frequency of these thoughts is the first step. Replacing them with more positive thoughts is the next.

Use the "Negative Thoughts Chart" at the end of the chapter and record your thoughts on it for as many days as you can. See how long it takes you to improve, what you still struggle with and how you think you can let go of the negativity. It will help you in other parts of your life as well.

EXCUSES, EXCUSES, EXCUSES

Excuses. Yes, words we have come up with to protect ourselves from fear, discomfort, guilt, or pain. The actual words mean nothing, but the underlying emotions mean everything. As we learned earlier, words can be powerful motivators in starting or stopping, or in adhering to or abandoning, an effective fitness program.

We all use excuses at one time or another. They serve us in the following ways:

1. **Denial.** A way to avoid dealing with the truth. An example might be to say, "I'm perfectly healthy," when that's not the case. Actually accepting that you may not be in good health—and could be cutting your life short—is a scary thought! It feels a lot better to pretend that possibility doesn't exist.

2. **Avoidance.** We use excuses to avoid confronting issues we are uncomfortable with. Perhaps we tell ourselves, "I don't have time right now," because we don't want to feel self-conscious walking into a gym.

3. **Rationalization.** A way to not feel guilty is to use excuses that provide logical explanations. Instead of admitting the truth—that you just don't want to exercise—you might say, "I've worked hard, it's the end of the week and I deserve a break today."

4. **Projection.** Using words to shift the blame onto someone else. This could be blaming a spouse as the reason you couldn't get up early enough. Maybe you felt you had to make them breakfast, take them to work, etc.

5. **Minimization.** Downplaying the importance of behavior. This might be an excuse, stating that you "only missed one week of working out; it's not a big deal."

Understand that these excuses serve to protect us, to preserve our self-esteem, and prevent us from feeling uncomfortable or fearful. But, over time, they can smother our personal growth and success at achieving our goals.

On the following "Facing My Fears" Worksheet, list the top five excuses you have used about why you don't exercise. List them all. Then go back and think about each one. What feeling or fear is each one covering up? Note that fear next to the excuse. When you're done listing all the excuses and how they serve to protect you, you should have a good idea of what you are trying NOT to feel. That's a critical step. By understanding what the feeling is, you can address it. You can deal with the fear directly. For example, the excuse might be, "I don't have enough time to work out – I'm too busy with home, kids and work." The fear? Will you feel inadequate? Maybe you risk being judged. Or are just downright afraid to change.

Reflect on how long the fear goes back. How have you handled that fear in other cases, over time? Have you found any ways to overcome it? Positive or negative? These are all important questions to ask, contemplate, and deal with so that you can relieve that underlying pain or fear. Once that immobilizing grip is gone, there won't be any need for the excuses. And adherence to your exercise plan will be so much easier.

Important: If you are dealing with deep trauma, you may need to seek help through a counselor, therapist, or other professional, and start journaling daily about your feelings. Talk more to friends and family about troubling issues. Once you have released the trauma and have learned how to handle it so it doesn't rule your life, you can move forward on your quest for fitness. You don't have to be pain-free to continue on this journey, but you do need to be aware of what is real and what is a coping mechanism used to protect you from pain.

So keep in the back of your mind: excuses are what we fall back on when we are afraid to take action. If you *really* want to do something, you will find a way to do it. Exercise doesn't have to cost money. If you're afraid of pain, remember it's a sign of overdoing it. Feeling self-conscious about being around others? Today, you can work out remotely without anyone even seeing you. If you truly don't know enough about exercise—what to do, which exercises are safe, how to set goals, or how to stay motivated—you're on your way with help. It's never too late, and there's always a way. Your biggest challenge will be to cut out the excuses and not give up on yourself! Starting now.

Move to the next page and start recording your negative thoughts on the "Negative Thoughts Chart." Then complete the "Facing My Fears" Worksheet that follows.

Negative Thoughts

Put a hash mark every time you have a negative thought. If it seems like a lot, no worries. This is about improvement over time.

MON	TUES	WED	THURS	FRI	SAT	SUN

Facing My Fears Worksheet

Objective: Use this worksheet to reflect on the reasons (excuses) you give for not exercising and identify the underlying feelings or fears associated with each excuse. This will help you understand what may be emotionally holding you back from succeeding in your fitness journey.

Step 1: List Your Excuses and Fears

In the table below, list all the excuses you can think of that you've used for not exercising. Be honest with yourself. Common excuses include lack of time, feeling too tired, fear of failure, etc.

Now, for each excuse, reflect on what feelings, emotions, or fears could be behind it. What is your excuse protecting you from? Examples might include fear of judgment, fear of failure, discomfort, or self-doubt. Write those feelings or fears next to the corresponding excuse.

Excuse	Underlying Feeling or Fear
1.	
2.	
3.	
4.	
5.	

Step 2: Reflect on the Impact of Your Fears

Take a moment to think about how these feelings or fears have impacted your fitness journey. How long have they been present? How have they influenced your decisions or behaviors? What would your fitness journey look like if these fears were addressed?

Use the space below to reflect:

Reflection:

_____

_____

Step 3: Moving Forward

Once you've identified your fears, think about how you can address them head-on. What steps can you take to release these fears or manage them in a healthier way? Are there specific actions or mindset shifts you can implement to overcome these emotional barriers?

Next Steps:

_____

_____

_____

_____

_____

_____

_____

_____

_____

Reminder: If you are dealing with deep emotional trauma or unresolved issues, you may need support from a counselor, therapist, or another professional. Acknowledging your fears is the first step to moving forward, but reaching out for help is sometimes necessary. You are not alone on this journey.

CHAPTER REFLECTION

Date: _____

What did I learn from this chapter?

What will I do differently or apply this week?

How do I feel after completing this chapter?

IN THE MOOD

What exactly is the definition of mood? It is a temporary emotional state or feeling that can affect a person's overall emotional state. Moods can change frequently and can last for minutes, hours, or days. When we say we 'aren't in the mood' to exercise or make healthy food choices, it's often a powerful feeling. This statement can encompass a variety of emotions—perhaps we're feeling fatigued, bored with our routine, or frustrated by our body image and expectations.

These moods can signal a deeper disconnection from our fitness goals. If our aspirations seem distant or unattainable, we might lean toward more immediate sources of pleasure, like indulging in comfort foods or skipping workouts. Understanding how our mood influences our motivation is crucial, as it serves as the foundation for making positive choices. In this chapter, we'll look at the intricate relationship between our mood and our commitment to healthier living, exploring how awareness of our emotional state can empower us to stay on track with our fitness journey.

Bottom line: Your mood significantly influences your exercise habits and motivation to eat healthily. When you're in a positive mood, you often feel more energized and motivated to stick to your exercise routine. Positive emotions enhance your confidence and self-efficacy, making it easier to believe you can achieve your fitness goals, which leads to greater adherence to exercise. The joy of movement can trigger the "runner's high," reinforcing your desire to work out regularly.

Conversely, negative moods can sap your motivation. When you're feeling down or stressed, you may lack the energy to work out, leading to skipped sessions or a reluctance to even get started. Low energy often fosters thoughts of self-sabotage, like "I can't do it" or "What's the point?" Additionally, during tough emotional moments, you might seek comfort in sedentary activities like binge-watching TV, which keeps you from engaging in physical activity.

Mood also plays a critical role in your eating choices. Negative feelings can lead to emotional eating, where food becomes a source of comfort rather than nourishment. This often results in unhealthy dietary choices, such as opting for junk food or overeating.

In contrast, when you're in a positive mood, you're more likely to make mindful eating decisions, focusing on the health benefits of what you consume. During these moments, you might naturally gravitate toward healthier options like fruits, vegetables, and whole grains, which can further enhance both your mood and physical health.

Interestingly, exercise itself can act as a mood enhancer. Physical activity releases endorphins, often called "feel-good hormones," which can elevate your spirits. Even if you start off feeling down, a workout can significantly improve your mental state, keeping you motivated for future exercise and healthier food choices.

The sense of accomplishment that comes from completing a workout also contributes to this positive cycle. It's essential to recognize how mood can create a cycle of reinforcement: a positive mood encourages exercise, which boosts mood further, while a negative mood can lead to less exercise, worsening your emotional state.

To navigate inevitable mood swings, having a strategy for those low-energy days is crucial. Consider opting for lighter workouts or incorporating gentler activities like yoga or walking to stay consistent without feeling overwhelmed. Embracing exercise as a therapeutic tool can also shift your perspective—view it as a means to improve your mood rather than solely relying on motivation. A quick walk or workout can be exactly what you need to lift your spirits, helping you maintain your commitment to fitness and healthy eating even when faced with emotional challenges.

Also, chart your feelings on the following "Mood Calendar". See how often you feel happy, sad, angry, afraid or confused and how that impacts the rest of your day. The chart will help you observe the relationship between your mood and your eating/activity routine. After a month, you will be able to see trends. Those trends, when brought to your awareness, will help you implement strategies to overcome negative feelings in a way that works for you.

For example, you notice that every Monday you are down and depressed. You don't want to exercise and you grab whatever food you see in sight. After thinking about it you realize that Monday is the most stressful day of the week for you. You're bombarded at work, have to get the kids out the door, plan dinner and you're tired before the day even starts. Strategies that could work to prevent that cycle would be to plan meals for that day ahead of time, bring the kids into your solution by having them help out or become part of your exercise that day. And adding some brief periods of mediation during the day could help as well.

Mood Calendar

Top half of each day indicates your general mood / bottom half indicates how well you stuck to exercise and a healthy eating pattern

MON	TUES	WED	THURS	FRI	SAT	SUN

Mood: Happy, Sad, Angry, Afraid, Confused

Exercise and Eating Pattern: Excellent, Good, Average, Not So Good, Poor

34

CHAPTER REFLECTION

Date: _____

What did I learn from this chapter?

What will I do differently or apply this week?

How do I feel after completing this chapter?

THE NUTRITION CONNECTION

NUTRITION BASICS

Food is important. You can follow everything in this book, set up the ideal program, and stick to it diligently—yet still not gain the results you hoped for. Why? Well, if we rule out genetics (which may also be a factor, but one we have no control over), the most likely snag is diet. What you eat is critical. So important that you could probably lose a great deal of body fat, look and feel much better by eating the right diet alone. Without one bit of exercise.

Of course you wouldn't want to leave out exercise, after all, you want all those verified benefits of exercise listed in the first part of the book. You want to be healthy both in mind and body. And prevent many of the diseases that come from inactivity.

Here's a common mistake: Have you ever exercised yourself to death, come home to pig out and then complain that your fitness program isn't working? If you drain a swimming pool at one end while you continue to fill it at the other, it's never going to empty. The same is true about fat. If you burn off fat only to continue to eat more of it, you won't be as successful at losing weight. The fat you eat is the same fat you work hard to burn off. If you want to get rid of fat, find realistic ways to reduce taking it in.

So if we reduce fat in our diets will that guarantee weight loss? It depends. If you take in an excess of any food, it will be converted to fat whether or not it contains any. Say you decide you're going to cut out eating potato chips. If you substitute a low fat food instead and eat fewer total calories you're most likely to lose weight. If, on the other hand, you substitute another low fat food but eat 10 times more calories you won't. Extra calories get stored as fat, regardless. Stay alert to the dangerous idea that you can eat more of an item just because it's lower in fat. That's just not true.

If you're not eating much fat, what should you be eating? Well, approximately two thirds of your diet should consist of carbohydrates. Yes, carbohydrates. They are not the villain. Carbohydrates are what give us instant energy and fuel our movements. Your brain won't function without them. The advantage you have when eating carbohydrates versus fats is that carbohydrates take more energy to be processed by the body than fat. So, you can burn a few more of them off. Make sure you eat mainly complex carbohydrates like whole grains, wheat bread, pasta, rice, cereals and high fiber foods instead of simple sugars found in candy and other goodies. The remaining third is divided between protein and fat - the less fat the better.

Usually consuming 10% of dietary fat is considered a "low-fat" diet and 30% or more high. Don't get hung up on keeping your intake of fat tremendously low, just pay attention to it and how much you're actually taking in. Aim for the 10% range. If you try to eliminate all fat you're asking for trouble. Body fat has important functions. It serves as an insulator, cushion, and is a stored energy source that is more abundant than any other.

As a rule of thumb, when reading a food label you should aim to choose foods that contain 3 grams or less of fat per every hundred calories. That means if you're aiming for a lower fat food a baked apple (approx.1 g per hundred calories) will be a better food choice than a slice of apple pie (approx. 5-8 g per hundred calories). You can also look at the entire meal that you're about to eat. If you're having several foods with no/low fat then one can have more fat in it – in this case it's the whole meal that you want to consider.

Once you start reading the food labels, especially on fast food, you will see the tremendous amount of fat included in our food supply. Just look at any of the cooking shows on TV. How many times do you see them start off with a stick of butter? Then add loads of cheese, cream or olive oil to the recipe. Sure, the recipe may look yummy but it's more suited to giving you heart disease. Especially if you eat like that every day.

If you like processed meats, like hot dogs, sandwich meats, and bacon, stop. Research has shown that these products are not only high in unhealthy fats but are also linked to a higher risk of cancer, especially colorectal cancer. The preservatives and chemicals used in processing—like nitrates and nitrites—are part of the reason they're so harmful.

What about protein? A healthy diet definitely needs enough protein. It's protein that is needed for hormones, enzymes, nails and hair. It works to heal, regenerate and is what all muscle and tissue is made out of. If you're one of those individuals who thinks you need extra protein because you're working out, that's not necessarily true. Only when you first start building muscle or develop a large amount of muscle mass will you need extra protein in your diet. Once you are fit, you don't need extra - it will only get broken down and flushed down the toilet anyway. Eliminating protein places extra strain on your kidneys. Protein supplements cannot provide energy (only carbohydrates or fat do) or guarantee that you'll become muscle-bound. So forget protein bars and shakes. They cost too much money and you don't need them. Protein is already in a lot of the food you eat daily. Eating massive amounts of protein to get more muscle doesn't work. Eating a sound diet in the right proportions and exercising is the best way to develop or add more definition to your body.

Alright, if you know what you should be eating and are giving it a good shot, just when should you eat? Before or after exercising? You can eat a light meal several hours before exercise for energy and performance. Make it mostly carbohydrate and a little bit of protein but low in fat. Bigger meals should be eaten after activity. When the stomach is full, blood is sent there for digestion and isn't available for working muscles. When you eat a huge meal and then exercise you may not be able to get much out of your muscles and end up feeling like a brick or worse yet, sick. So, stick with something light (like toast or a peanut butter sandwich) if you're going to eat beforehand and make it several hours in advance.

There are plenty of books and information on nutrition and diet. Eat foods that have high nutritional value vs. empty calories. Read through the following "Nutritional Value" list of foods for examples. It should help you learn how to differentiate between nutritious, healthy plant-based foods vs those that are void of adequate nutritional benefits. The high nutritional value foods are nutrient-rich, minimally processed, and offer a variety of vitamins, minerals, and fiber. They fill you up faster and keep you full longer. Low nutritional value foods tend to be highly processed and contain added sugars, unhealthy fats, and artificial ingredients.

As far as vitamins and minerals go, if you eat a good diet you probably won't need extra in the form of supplements. If you're not sure though, it wouldn't hurt to take some type of multiple vitamin/mineral supplement. Mega doses of vitamins will not boost performance or energy level. Energy comes from food - not vitamins. If you take vitamins be sure to take them with your meals so that they actually get absorbed. When you take them alone they are useless - you may as well dump them in the toilet instead. Other pills and potions are on the market which promise boundless energy and higher metabolism. Beware! None of these products have been proven to do anything by themselves. The fine print always reads something to the effect of "...for best results must be used in conjunction with a healthy diet and regular exercise." Whenever you see this it tells you that the diet and exercise is what really does the trick, not the bogus product.

NUTRITIONAL VALUE OF COMMON FOODS

High Nutritional Value	Low Nutritional Value
Leafy greens (spinach, kale, arugula)	French fries
Berries (blueberries, strawberries, raspberries)	Soda and sugary drinks
Lentils, black beans, and chickpeas	White bread
Quinoa, farro, and bulgur	Packaged chips
Sweet potatoes and yams	Candy and sweets
Almonds, walnuts, cashews	Sugary cereals
Avocado	Instant noodles
Edamame, green peas	Frozen pizza
Broccoli, cauliflower, Brussels sprouts	White rice
Mushrooms (portobello, cremini, shiitake)	Fried snacks
Chia seeds, sunflower seeds	Ice cream
Whole grains (brown rice, oats, barley)	Highly processed granola bars
Carrots, beets, and parsnips	Crackers
Zucchini, squash	Processed cheese slices
Tofu and tempeh	Packaged snack cakes
Bell peppers, tomatoes	Sweetened yogurt
Cucumbers, celery	Sweetened nut milks
Apples, pears, oranges	Canned fruit in syrup
Bananas, grapes	Chips and salsa
Green beans, snap peas	Pop-Tarts
Hummus and bean dips	Energy drinks

High Nutritional Value	Low Nutritional Value
Spinach, Swiss chard	Canned soup (high sodium)
Fresh herbs (basil, parsley, cilantro)	Frosted pastries
Whole grain bread	Sugary granola
Cabbage and Bok choy	Candy bars
Pomegranate and citrus fruits	Frozen French toast sticks
Nuts and dried fruit (unsweetened)	Sugary pancake mix
Oatmeal (unsweetened)	Cookies
Radishes, turnips	Processed snack bars

When choosing foods that are not on this list, guess which category the food would be placed in. If it's a better fit for the low nutritional column, best to opt for a better choice.

YOUR DIET

If you happen to be an emotional eater (that is one who eats in response to feelings instead of hunger) you may want to take it one step further. Fill out the food ledger which follows. It consists of a food diary to record all food and liquid taken in for three days, two weekdays, and one weekend. Categories for amounts eaten and calorie counts of each food are also included. Plus a place to list what you were doing while eating, the time of day, how well you liked a specific food, and how hungry you were when you ate it.

After you complete the ledger you'll see how many calories you're eating each day. Women typically need around 1,800–2,200 calories per day, while men often need about 2,200–2,800, depending on their age, size, and activity level. You'll also be able to see trends such as eating during a specific time of day or during a certain activity. Key in on foods you eat simply because you like the taste of them, not because you're hungry (which means you're feeding something other than hunger).

Use the information you've entered to see how you can make tiny steps towards healthier eating. After you've completed the food ledger you'll see a guide called "Tips on Changing Your Eating Habits". It will help you start the thought process on some simple changes that you can make on your own. Choose just one item to work on at a time. For example, if you love ice cream, freeze several bananas that are cut into small pieces. Blend them in a food processor until you have what is called "nice cream." It's a great substitute and you can add flavorings like vanilla. Once that has become a new habit, move on to the next one. Give yourself time for each change, at least a month or two to really solidify your new routine.

The food ledger can be a valuable tool to use too when you seek the aid of a nutritionist or therapist. They'll be able to spot details you may not notice on your own and help you even further. So, take the time to fill it out, even if it sits around for a while or you aren't sure how to interpret it. As long as it reflects your current eating behavior you can use it later if you feel the need to see either of the above professionals.

The main point, eat a sensible diet low in fat and devoid of overly processed foods. Too much of anything can get turned into unwanted fat. If you feel out of control when it comes to food get help from a qualified professional, otherwise your weight loss efforts may suffer.

WEIGHT MANAGEMENT FOOD LEDGER

Please fill in everything you eat and drink for the next 5 days (do not mix and match days). Make sure one of the days is a Saturday or Sunday. It is important that you eat exactly the same as you would normally. In fact, calculate the calories, carbohydrates, fat, and protein grams **AFTER** the five days. This must be a true representation of how and what you usually eat.

Here is what you need to put in each column:

- **Column #1:** Write in the food eaten/liquid consumed.

- **Column #2:** Indicate amount (cups, ounces, tbsp., etc.).

- **Column #3:** Indicate where you were or what you were doing (e.g., in the car, watching TV, lunch at work, at a party, etc.).

- **Column #4:** Rate on a scale from 0-5 how hungry you were (0 = not hungry, 5 = starving).

- **Column #5:** Rate how much you liked the food from 0-5 (0 = don't care for the food, 5 = love the food, a favorite).

- **Column #6:** Total fat grams in the food.

- **Column #7:** Total protein grams in the food.

- **Column #8:** Total carbohydrate grams in the food.

- **Column #9:** Total calories in the food.

Use package nutrient information, fast food nutritional charts (usually posted, or ask), or check online to estimate calories, fat, protein, and carbohydrates.

Remember, be honest and eat as you usually would. In order to make positive changes, you must know precisely what is happening with what you eat. It may even be tedious or embarrassing logging in everything, but it will help you in the long run to change your eating habits for the better.

Make copies of the actual ledger on the next page so that you have 1-2 copies per day to enter your foods on.

FOOD LEDGER

FOOD/DRINK	AMOUNT	WHERE	HUNGER	LIKE	FAT (g)	CARBS (g)	PROTEIN (g)	KCALS

Duplicate pages before entering information, you will need several pages

Tips on Changing Your Eating Habits

1. If You're Eating Too Many Calories:

- **Portion Control:** Try using smaller plates and serving sizes to help reduce your calorie intake without feeling deprived.
- **Eat Mindfully:** Slow down while eating to allow your body time to recognize when it's full. Avoid distractions like TV or smartphones during meals.
- **Track Snacks:** Watch out for high-calorie snacks. Replace chips or sweets with lower-calorie alternatives like fruits, vegetables, or nuts in moderation.

2. If You're Eating Too Many Non-Nutritious Foods:

- **Add More Whole Foods:** Incorporate more whole grains, lean proteins, fruits, and vegetables. Focus on nutrient-dense options like leafy greens, berries, and beans.
- **Swap Unhealthy Ingredients:** Replace refined grains (white bread, pasta) with whole grains and opt for healthier cooking methods like baking or steaming instead of frying.
- **Plan Balanced Meals:** Aim for meals that include a balance of protein, healthy fats, and fiber-rich carbohydrates to help keep you full and satisfied.

3. If You're Eating For Emotional Reasons:

- **Identify Triggers:** Keep a journal of when and why you emotionally eat. Recognizing stress, boredom, or anxiety as triggers helps you address them without turning to food.
- **Find Alternatives:** When you feel emotional cravings, try a different coping mechanism like going for a walk, journaling, or talking to a friend instead of eating.
- **Practice Stress Management:** Incorporate stress-relief techniques like meditation, deep breathing, or exercise into your daily routine to reduce emotional eating.

4. If You're Eating Just Because You Like the Taste:

- **Moderation is Key:** It's okay to enjoy your favorite foods but try to keep portions reasonable. Savor them by eating slowly and mindfully.
- **Balance Indulgences:** If you're eating something you enjoy but that isn't nutritious, balance it out with healthier meals throughout the day.
- **Limit Temptations:** Keep indulgent, less nutritious foods out of sight or out of your home to reduce temptation or save them for special occasions instead of

daily consumption. If you feel you can't control yourself around them, don't buy them!

5. Tips for Eating a Balanced Diet:

- **Include All Food Groups:** Aim to incorporate a variety of foods from all major food groups—fruits, vegetables, whole grains, lean proteins, and healthy fats—into your meals each day. This ensures you get a range of essential nutrients.
- **Eat Colorfully:** A good rule of thumb is to "eat the rainbow" by choosing fruits and vegetables of different colors. Each color offers different vitamins and minerals, such as red tomatoes (rich in lycopene), orange carrots (high in beta-carotene), and green spinach (packed with iron and calcium). For optimal health you need 9 servings a day.
- **Balance Macronutrients:** Every meal should include a balance of macronutrients:
  - **Protein**: Include beans, tofu, or legumes to support muscle growth and repair.
  - **Healthy Fats**: Choose avocado, nuts, seeds and olive oil for heart health.
  - **Complex Carbohydrates**: Go for whole grains like brown rice, quinoa, oats, and sweet potatoes for sustained energy.
- **Control Portion Sizes:** Avoid overloading on any single food group. Half your plate should consist of vegetables and fruits, with the other half divided between protein and whole grains.
- **Stay Hydrated:** Water plays an essential role in digestion and overall health. Make sure to drink water throughout the day and include water-rich foods like cucumbers, watermelon, and leafy greens. Thirst is often mistaken for hunger. Drink a glass of water before meals and throughout the day to stay hydrated.
- **Limit Processed Foods:** Minimize your intake of highly processed foods, which are often high in unhealthy fats, sugars, and sodium. Instead, focus on whole, minimally processed foods. This includes hot dogs, sandwich meat and bacon.
- **Plan Ahead:** Prepare balanced meals and snacks ahead of time to ensure you stay on track with a healthy diet, especially during busy days. Meal prepping can help you avoid relying on less nutritious, convenient options.
- **Listen to Your Body:** Learn to recognize true hunger and fullness signals, which can help prevent overeating. Aim to eat when you're genuinely hungry and stop when you're satisfied, not overly full.

CHAPTER REFLECTION

Date: _____

What did I learn from this chapter?

What will I do differently or apply this week?

How do I feel after completing this chapter?

WHAT'S UP, DOC?

Everyone's heard it yet tries to avoid the standard warning — get the OK from your physician BEFORE you begin to exercise. Yes, it may seem like a hassle to make an appointment and go to the doctor, especially if there's nothing apparently wrong with you. Maybe you don't particularly get along well with your physician and don't relish the idea of talking about your weight or exercise. If that's the case, now's the time to find another doctor.

I've heard many people tell me their doctor didn't want them to do aerobic exercise yet gave no sound medical reason why. Then, the same doctor turns around and gives them a list of exercises that have been contraindicated for the past decade. Don't expect your doctor to know much about exercise except that it's good for you. As stated before, only 24% of adults in this country regularly exercise enough to benefit themselves. The chances of your doctor being one of the 24% are not too likely. Ask what type of aerobic and strength exercise they do and see. Hobbies and games like playing golf and gardening don't count.

A physician's specialty is disease and medicine. You need a doctor to provide medical clearance so that you know you are healthy enough to begin an exercise program. They don't have the knowledge to give you an exercise program. They have not been trained in that field. I have personally gone to doctors who have given me exercises that are outdated, unsafe or plain ineffective. A reminder that their training is in medicine, not in prescribing movement. One of my previous students went to her doctor because she had a frozen shoulder (couldn't lift her arm above shoulder level). Her doctor had this advice: "If you can't lift your arm above your head, don't do that." Well that wasn't going to do her any good. But a routine of icing, stretching and strengthening did. Bottom line, doctors should be consulted for medical issues, not exercise selection.

There are many conditions that may make it necessary for you to have a specialized program developed just for you, BUT always remember, if you're alive, you can exercise. No matter what limitation you're faced with, there are ways to help you become more fit and healthy. If you have known heart disease, you may need specialized routines different from those suitable for the general population. Still, there's no reason why you can't get started and gradually increase your endurance and strength. When I owned my studio, I had a student who was over 50, with dangerously high cholesterol, on several medications, and who had triple bypass surgery. He did classes with my most advanced group and biked on the off days. He was resolved to staying fit. If he can do it, so can you — if you get started the right way.

Maybe unbeknownst to you, you have heart disease, hypertension, diabetes, or abnormal blood cholesterol levels. You need a doctor to uncover these conditions so that you can take necessary precautions. Maybe you'll need medication to increase safety during physical activity. Regardless, you want to know what your physical condition is and what you need to be cautious of. Say you have something more serious like loss of a limb, severe back trauma, or crippling arthritis. No, you won't be running marathons next month, but you can still find a way to be more fit tomorrow than you are today. If you blindly start a fitness routine, get into it, and then discover you have a serious problem, you may have to discontinue your program or drastically alter it.

In some cases, exercise may make the problem worse. For example, say you have a structural problem with your feet and start a running program. Months later, you're in pain, can hardly walk, let alone run, and have to stop exercising. You go to your doctor to find out that you have a condition that could be remedied by wearing orthotics. After several weeks off to recuperate, you finally get the orthotics and start your program again. This time, you change the routine to a brisk walk, feel great, have no problems, and don't miss days because you're in pain. Seeing your doctor first could have prevented a lot of agony and time off.

If you already have specific muscle or joint disorders, definitely seek the advice of a chiropractor too. They specialize in how muscles and bones work together with the nervous system and can offer you many insights a medical doctor isn't trained to give.

You also want to know what effect any medication you're taking may have on your heart rate during exercise. Some medications (diet pills, amphetamines, nicotine) elevate your working heart rate, others (beta blockers) lower it, and many vary widely in their effects based on time taken and dosage (like calcium channel blockers and antihypertensives). Even if you're on a slew of medications, that's no excuse not to work out. It's just more important for you and/or your exercise leader to know about all medications you're on and design your program around them.

Youth doesn't necessarily protect you from risk factors either. Everyone should seek the approval of a physician before starting their program. Anyone who has been sedentary for any length of time, is closer to 50 than 20, is pregnant, or who has family members with heart disease, should be even more adamant about physician approval. Even though a doctor can't tell you what specific exercises you should do for your situation, he or she can tell you whether or not it's safe for you to work your muscles (including the heart) at this moment in time. Whatever the prognosis is, keep a positive outlook. As long as you can move, you can get fit. There are hundreds of ways to exercise and have fun doing it.

The key message here — go to your doctor! If you don't have one, don't proceed any further until you find one you absolutely like and trust. Find someone you feel you can talk to and discuss questions with. Someone who is on the same wavelength as you and whom you're likely to believe. And someone who gives you the impression they care about you as a person and not simply the 10 minutes of time you're scheduled to fill.

In addition to seeing the doctor, fill out the health history form that follows. Use it later when working with a personal trainer or exercise leader. If you don't have either, you can still use it to learn more about what exercises are potentially hazardous for you and which are especially important as well.

If you checked "YES" to any of the questions, mark the page so you can come back later or make a copy to keep handy for the rest of the reading. The more health conditions you list the more important it is for you to take steps to get fit now. Before something catastrophic happens.

HEALTH HISTORY FORM

Name:

_____

Age: _____ Gender: _____ Date: _____

Physician's Name: _____ Phone #: _____

Does your physician know you are starting an exercise program?
If yes, does he/she advise it? _____

Emergency Contact:_____ Phone #: _____

In the past three months:

1. Have you been on any medication?

    _____

2. Have you been or are you currently pregnant?

    _____

3. Have you been completely sedentary?
    If not, what activity have you been doing?

    _____

Do you have (or had within the past year):

1. Heart problems

    _____

2. Heart problems in the family

    _____

3. High blood pressure

    _____

4. High blood cholesterol

_____

5. Surgery

_____

6. Obesity

_____

7. Diabetes

_____

8. Lung problems

_____

9. Cigarette smoking habit

_____

10. A chronic illness

_____

11. Difficulty with physical exertion

_____

12. Back, knee, or other muscle/joint problems

_____

CHAPTER REFLECTION

Date: _____

What did I learn from this chapter?

What will I do differently or apply this week?

How do I feel after completing this chapter?

ACTIVITY SELECTION

Once you've gotten the go-ahead from your doctor, you're ready to choose your activity. The type of activity that will work best for you depends upon several factors.

First, you'll want to make sure you actually have a program that will be effective at improving your health and fitness level. Then, narrow down the selection according to your goals, restrictions, and what you consider 'fun' to do. Choosing the right activity can assure you of enjoyment, results, and an enduring plan. Choosing the wrong activity can set you up to bail before you even begin.

Before starting the selection process, keep in mind that there are four basic components to physical fitness. Ignore one, and you won't achieve balanced health. They are: 1) muscular strength 2) muscular endurance 3) cardiovascular endurance and 4) flexibility.

Muscular strength is important because strong, developed muscles lead to a boosted metabolic rate, even when you aren't working out. That means you will burn more calories even at rest. Having strong muscles also prevents you from sustaining many injuries and is responsible for the sculpted look so many people strive for. To develop strength, you must perform movements against a resistance—either from your own body weight (like a push-up) or through the use of resistance products (weights, tubing, etc.). This is called "anaerobic" exercise.

Muscular endurance refers to how long a specific muscle can perform a move without getting tired. Increasing muscular endurance can lead to less overall fatigue and make simple things—like climbing stairs or walking to the store—more enjoyable and comfortable to do. To develop endurance, the same movements are repeated over and over again, gradually increasing the number performed. For example, walking builds endurance of specific leg muscles through repeated motion. Over time, endurance gains are demonstrated by the ability to complete longer and longer walks.

Cardiovascular endurance is the ability of the heart and lung system to deliver blood to the rest of the body. A stronger cardiopulmonary system offers protection against premature diseases of the heart, blood vessels, and lungs. To increase cardiovascular endurance or aerobic capacity, you need to do some type of "aerobic" exercise. Aerobic exercise uses the large muscles in the legs repeatedly and continuously to strengthen the cardiovascular system. When working aerobically, you'll feel your body get warmer, your heart rate goes up, and your breathing rate increases. Examples are brisk walking, running, biking, swimming, stepping, etc. Aerobic exercise is also the only type of exercise that burns fat as a source of fuel, so it is necessary to include it in programs for fat loss.

Flexibility is the ability of the muscles to stretch, which allows your joints to move through a greater range of motion. Children have great flexibility but generally lose it by adulthood if not exposed to stretching. Flexibility is important in preventing injury. It helps runners take a longer stride. It also makes movement in general more comfortable and easy. The best way to stay limber and flexible is to stretch muscles to their longest comfortable position and stay there for 30-60 seconds. For example, to stretch your chest muscles, bring your arms behind you, clasp your hands, lift, and hold.

To ensure you are improving your total health and well-being, you need to include a segment of your workout to address each of these areas. For example, you could go for a walk for aerobics and endurance, return to do strength work for arms and legs, and finish with stretching. All of the above four components are included— so your program is balanced. If, however, you walk only and don't do the other exercises for strength and flexibility, your program is not balanced, and you're depriving yourself of the benefits the other parts can offer.

Tailor your program to your specific situation; that is, address each of the four areas but place the emphasis on the areas that are most directly associated with your goals. For example, if you want to lose fat, spend more time on aerobic exercise and strength work, and less time on flexibility. If you're recovering from serious back problems, focus more heavily on stretching and strengthening than aerobics. If you are the average sedentary person who just hasn't done anything for years, balance the four out. Aim for at least 20 minutes of aerobics, strengthening exercises that target all the major muscles, and 5-10 minutes of stretching each time.

You may have to combine different activities to balance your workout. For example, golfing would need to be combined with strength and flexibility exercises to be considered a total body workout. Even then, you may have to do additional continuous aerobic activity to improve cardiovascular fitness. If you don't have the time to do all these things, don't choose golf as your fitness activity. It's considered more of a game than actual exercise.

NARROWING DOWN THE CHOICES

Go back to Chapter 3 and revisit what you put down as reasons why you want to exercise. Do you want to lose weight? Is it because your doctor told you to? Maybe you want to get some definition in those muscles. Or perhaps you want to control chronic pain or an illness like diabetes. It's absolutely important that you know why you are doing this in the first place before you start!

Foremost, if you don't know what your goals are, you won't know how to achieve them. For example, if you want to exercise to lose weight, you know you must do aerobic exercise and strength training. Enrolling in a yoga class is not going to accomplish that, no matter how long you do it. If you suffer from chronic pain, however, yoga combined with light aerobic activity like walking or swimming would be ideal. Your goals need to be matched with activities that will help you safely reach them.

RESTRICTIONS

Be realistic about limitations—we all have them. If you're older and haven't worked out for a good number of years, running is probably not going to be a good choice for you to start with, but walking or spinning classes would be fine. Maybe you're overweight to the point of being obese. Riding a bike or playing tennis may be just too uncomfortable to do. Instead, choose walking, light aerobic classes, or water activities. Be mindful of anything that can undermine your ability to perform your routine.

It may be you don't have much time. If that's the case, don't expect to do your activity every single day, or you'll be let down when you can't fit it in. If you live 30 minutes away from the health club you're thinking of joining, chances are you're not going to drive there often enough to benefit.

You know yourself better than anyone else. Think realistically about what you're willing to do and what you know won't last. Work your program around your particular boundaries so they never become an excuse for abandoning the program.

GETTING MOTIVATED

Intrinsic vs. Extrinsic Motivation

If you don't mind being alone, are disciplined, and find activity personally satisfying, you're likely internally motivated—or 'intrinsic." On the other hand, if you find it extremely difficult to stay excited and dedicated to activities without having group support, interaction, and external rewards, then you can deem yourself extrinsically motivated or "extrinsic." Although most people usually fall into both categories, one will predominate. The workout program you choose can be doomed to failure if you don't take this point into consideration.

For example, someone primarily intrinsically motivated will have little problem maintaining a consistent exercise program at home alone. Workout apps, walking, exercise machines, and other workout equipment in the home can easily be managed out of the sheer enjoyment and internal drive of the person. For the extrinsic person, the same workout design can be disastrous. To maintain a regular routine, the extrinsic person needs to find an activity that will be rewarding through other benefits, such as making new friends, joking around, earning recognition from others, etc.

Many of us don't do very well on our own and may be considered extrinsic. What's going on around us is more important than the activity itself. Extrinsically motivated people may lose motivation early in their workout regime if they've chosen the wrong activity. So, think about this when you select what you plan on doing regularly. Regardless of whether you're intrinsic or extrinsic, there are ways to capitalize on both types of motivation.

First, make sure your workout contains an intrinsic factor by making it something you truly like. What do you consider fun? It's simple—if you hate biking, don't do it. If you loathe running, that's out. If you don't thoroughly enjoy the mode of exercise, it won't last. Think about all the activities available to you. There's walking, swimming, aerobic classes, boxing, martial arts, country line dancing, ballroom dancing, weightlifting, skiing, skating, yoga, street dancing, step aerobics, sliding, chair aerobics, ballet, jazz, modern dance, soccer, tennis, volleyball, basketball, gymnastics, wrestling, hockey, sledding, horseback riding, water polo, surfing, rugby, handball, racquetball, fencing, etc., etc., etc. The possibilities are really numerous if you take some time and think about it.

It's vital to pick something you would really enjoy doing on a regular basis. What kinds of activities did you love growing up? Which activities have special significance to you? Choose a movement or combination of various movements that you sincerely like. If you didn't have any, what types of activities spark your curiosity? Pick something you are at least somewhat interested in. Then, when you get deeper into the workout program, you'll be able to fall back on your enjoyment of the activity to keep you involved. Build in positive reinforcers too, like keeping track of each workout session you do. By looking at a graph and seeing on paper how many times you've already exercised, you'll be more encouraged to continue.

To boost extrinsic motivation, find a way to make your routine involve others. Join a club, class, or other group that meets regularly. Exchange phone numbers with several other people so that you can rely on them for support. Get involved in friendly contests or games. That way, at times when you lack the internal drive, the other benefits you get from the workout (friends, social outings outside of class, awards, etc.) may be just enough to keep you on track.

Regardless of whether you're designing your own program or entering a structured one, you must keep the above components of fitness in mind and work around your goals, restrictions, and motivational mode. If you plan on joining a club or facility, check out all the classes you'll take before joining.

You'll find an "Exercise Suggestion Guide" on the next page to help give you an idea of which category of exercises would be appropriate for a number of individual circumstances. Slowly work your way through the worksheet and finish before going any further. Even if you don't know what strength exercises are or which stretches you need to do, still identify which types of exercise you want in your plan. You'll get detailed sample plans later to help you get started. You have the power to choose what you do. Identifying what needs to be in your exercise routine will help ensure you reach your fitness goals.

EXERCISE SUGGESTION GUIDE

1. Arthritic

- **Strength:** Resistance bands, light weights, aquatic exercises.
- **Endurance:** Walking, cycling, swimming.
- **Cardio:** Low-impact aerobics, stationary bike.
- **Flexibility:** Gentle yoga, stretching, tai chi.

2. Asthmatic

- **Strength:** Bodyweight exercises, resistance training with controlled breathing.
- **Endurance:** Walking, swimming (humid environment helps breathing), cycling.
- **Cardio:** Moderate-intensity activities like brisk walking or stationary biking.
- **Flexibility:** Gentle stretching, yoga with a focus on breath control.

3. Back Pain

- **Strength:** Core strengthening exercises (e.g., planks, bridges), water therapy.
- **Endurance:** Walking, elliptical machine, recumbent bike.
- **Cardio:** Low-impact aerobics, swimming.
- **Flexibility:** Pilates, yoga focused on lower back stretches, gentle stretching.

4. Basic Couch Potato

- **Strength:** Bodyweight exercises (e.g., squats, wall push-ups), resistance bands.
- **Endurance:** Walking, light jogging, dance workouts.
- **Cardio:** Beginner-friendly cardio workouts like dancing, brisk walking.

- **Flexibility:** Simple stretching routines, yoga for beginners.

5. Bursitis/Tendinitis

- **Strength:** Isometric exercises, water-based resistance exercises.
- **Endurance:** Cycling, swimming, elliptical.
- **Cardio:** Low-impact activities to avoid joint irritation.
- **Flexibility:** Gentle stretching, range-of-motion exercises.

6. Heart Disease

- **Strength:** Light weightlifting, resistance bands under medical supervision.
- **Endurance:** Walking, stationary biking.
- **Cardio:** Cardiac rehabilitation-approved activities like brisk walking.
- **Flexibility:** Stretching exercises, tai chi.

7. Children

- **Strength:** Fun bodyweight exercises (e.g., jumping jacks, climbing).
- **Endurance:** Running, playing sports, biking.
- **Cardio:** Swimming, dancing, active play.
- **Flexibility:** Stretching, gymnastics, dance-based stretches.

8. Chronically Ill

- **Strength:** Light resistance training, bodyweight exercises.
- **Endurance:** Walking, swimming, cycling (if able).
- **Cardio:** Low-impact aerobics, stationary bike.
- **Flexibility:** Gentle stretching, yoga, chair yoga.

9. Diabetic

- **Strength:** Resistance bands, weight training.

- **Endurance:** Brisk walking, swimming, cycling.
- **Cardio:** Moderate aerobic activities (e.g., dancing).
- **Flexibility:** Stretching, yoga, Pilates.

10. Disabled

- **Strength:** Adaptive resistance training, bodyweight exercises.
- **Endurance:** Adaptive sports, hand cycling, seated aerobics.
- **Cardio:** Chair-based cardio workouts, seated boxing.
- **Flexibility:** Stretching, chair yoga, tai chi.

11. Emphysema/Bronchitis

- **Strength:** Resistance exercises with controlled breathing.
- **Endurance:** Walking, swimming.
- **Cardio:** Low-intensity exercises like walking or stationary bike.
- **Flexibility:** Gentle stretching, yoga focusing on breath control.

12. Epilepsy

- **Strength:** Weight training with supervision.
- **Endurance:** Walking, swimming, cycling.
- **Cardio:** Low-impact cardio workouts.
- **Flexibility:** Stretching, yoga.

13. Injured

- **Strength:** Isometric exercises, resistance bands, rehab exercises.
- **Endurance:** Walking, swimming, stationary cycling.
- **Cardio:** Low-impact activities like aqua jogging.
- **Flexibility:** Gentle stretching, rehab-specific yoga.

14. Knee Problems

- **Strength:** Leg lifts, water-based exercises, resistance bands.
- **Endurance:** Cycling, swimming.
- **Cardio:** Low-impact aerobics, elliptical.
- **Flexibility:** Gentle stretching, yoga focused on knee health.

15. Obese

- **Strength:** Bodyweight exercises, resistance bands, light weights.
- **Endurance:** Walking, water aerobics, biking.
- **Cardio:** Low-impact activities like swimming or walking.
- **Flexibility:** Chair yoga, stretching, tai chi.

16. Older Adult

- **Strength:** Resistance bands, light weight training.
- **Endurance:** Walking, swimming, cycling.
- **Cardio:** Low-impact aerobics, walking.
- **Flexibility:** Chair yoga, stretching, tai chi.

17. Postpartum/Nursing Woman

- **Strength:** Bodyweight exercises, light weight training.
- **Endurance:** Walking, swimming.
- **Cardio:** Low-impact aerobic exercises.
- **Flexibility:** Postnatal yoga, gentle stretching.

18. Pregnant

- **Strength:** Prenatal strength training, resistance bands.
- **Endurance:** Walking, swimming.
- **Cardio:** Low-impact aerobics, water aerobics.
- **Flexibility:** Prenatal yoga, stretching.

19. Smoker

- **Strength:** Bodyweight exercises, resistance training.
- **Endurance:** Walking, cycling, swimming.
- **Cardio:** Moderate-intensity cardio activities.
- **Flexibility:** Stretching, yoga.

20. Visually Impaired

- **Strength:** Bodyweight exercises, resistance bands.
- **Endurance:** Tandem cycling, swimming.
- **Cardio:** Adaptive sports, walking.
- **Flexibility:** Yoga, stretching exercises with guidance.

If none of the above apply to you, feel free to choose what you like for the four components of fitness.

At the end of the book, there are ready made strength and stretching routines if you prefer to simply follow a pre-formulated plan that safely targets all the major muscles. Then, you will only need to add an aerobic component and you're good to go!

CHAPTER REFLECTION

Date: _____

What did I learn from this chapter?

What will I do differently or apply this week?

How do I feel after completing this chapter?

THE HEART OF THE MATTER

When you drive a car, you monitor your speed to ensure you're going fast enough to reach your destination but not so fast that you risk bigger problems like a ticket or an accident. Monitoring your heart rate during exercise works the same way. If you're working below your capabilities, you won't make the progress you're aiming for—you'll just be wasting time. But if you push too hard, you risk injury or burnout, preventing you from reaching your goals safely. That's why it's crucial to know how much effort you're putting in during exercise.

The best way to make sure your exercise program is doable is to monitor your heart rate. There are several ways to figure out how hard your heart should be working, but first, let's go over some key terms:

Maximal Heart Rate: The highest your heart rate should ever reach. It's estimated by subtracting your age from 220.

Resting Heart Rate: The number of beats per minute when you're at complete rest. The best time to take this is first thing in the morning, before you even get out of bed. As your fitness improves, your resting heart rate should drop. A lower resting heart rate means your heart is becoming more efficient at pumping blood, which helps protect against heart disease.

To find your resting heart rate, count the beats on your wrist for one full minute in the morning. A typical resting heart rate ranges from 55-75 beats per minute (BPM), while anything above 100 BPM is considered high.

Target Heart Rate: This is how hard your heart should be working during exercise to see benefits. It's also called your working or training heart rate.

Target Heart Rate Zone: The specific range where you want your heart rate to be during exercise. The lower end is for when you're starting out, and the higher end is where you'll aim as your fitness improves. Later, you'll calculate your own Target Heart Rate Zone using the Karvonen method.

Recovery Heart Rate: This measures how quickly your heart returns to normal after exercise. A faster recovery indicates a stronger heart. The bigger the drop between your working heart rate and your recovery heart rate, the better.

THREE HEART RATE MEASUREMENT METHODS

1. **Perceived Exertion**: This is just how hard you realize the exercise to be. A perceived exertion scale goes from either 6 - 20 or 1 - 10. Either way, the low end of the scale represents little or no exertion, while the high end represents very, very hard or maximal exertion. To use the perceived exertion method simply go by how you feel. Do you feel as if you are exerting yourself? How much? You need to work to a point at which you feel the exercise is fairly light to somewhat hard. After you are exercising for a while you can increase the intensity but stay at the light end for a bit, until you get into the routine and realize you won't die. Usually perceived exertion is used along with the calculated method above. It is possible to think you're working harder than you actually are. In the same way, you may think you're not working hard enough. Perceived exertion is easy to use but for best results, use it with another method.

2. **Talk Test:** Another simple way to gauge intensity is to see if you can carry on a conversation during exercise. If you're pushing so hard you can't talk, you're working too hard. You should feel heavier breathing but still be able to talk without gasping for air.

3. **Karvonen Method:** My favorite way to calculate heart rate. Let's say you have three people of the same age, but with different fitness levels: one who's sedentary, one who exercises occasionally, and one who's a marathon runner. Obviously, these three people will need different levels of intensity in their workouts. A generic heart rate chart at the gym, which

only considers age, won't be accurate for them. That's why it's essential to calculate your own individual target heart rate—using the Karvonen method.

First, you need to know how to take your pulse; you can feel it at your wrist, neck, temple, or chest. On the wrist, it's just below the base of the thumb on the palm side of your arm. At the neck, it's below the jawline between the ear and the center of the throat. On the temple, it's above the eyebrows, and for the chest, you can place your entire hand over your heart. Remember to use your fingers, not your thumb, to avoid counting your thumb's pulse. Of course if you have a smart watch, the device will tell you your pulse rate but it's still important to know how to calculate it yourself.

Practice finding your pulse in these areas until you can reliably feel it. If you carry excess fat, it might be harder to find your pulse, so practice more often until you can count it accurately. It's best to use the wrist or neck (radial or carotid arteries) for exercise, but I prefer the wrist because it's safer. If you press too hard on the carotid artery, you risk cutting off blood flow to the brain, which could cause you to pass out—especially if there's blockage on the other side of your neck, you're older or have medical issues.

When taking your pulse, keep moving slightly. Stopping suddenly during intense exercise can make you dizzy. Count your pulse for 10 seconds to get an accurate measure. Then, use the formula at the end of the chapter to determine your target heart rate by plugging in your resting heart rate, age, and doing some basic math.

As your fitness level improves, you may find that it takes more effort to elevate your heart rate. When starting out, aim for around 60% of your target heart rate to avoid burning out too quickly. As you get fitter, you can gradually increase your intensity, eventually reaching the higher end of your target range. At that point, consider using 85% of your target heart rate as your new goal.

Remember, working above this level isn't necessary for maximizing calorie burn. At higher intensities, your body may rely more on other fuel sources rather than tapping into fat stores and carbohydrates. While high-intensity interval training (HIIT) workouts can be popular and challenging, they don't necessarily provide additional benefits compared to moderate-intensity workouts. Moreover, if you're not adequately conditioned, such strenuous exercises can increase the risk of injury. Doing less than what you are capable of, at least when beginning, is preferable than doing too much.

Eventually, you may not even need to take your pulse. You'll know your body well enough to sense when you're working at the right intensity. But while you're starting out, tracking your heart rate is the best way to ensure you're doing enough without overdoing it.

Use the calculation sheet at the end of this section to figure out your own target heart rate. You'll need your age and your heart rate while you are at complete rest. Then just plug the numbers into the sheet to see what your working heart rate should range from. There is an example provided after the calculation page just in case you need additional help to do the math.

As you get older and more fit, your age and resting rate change so you'll need to recalculate periodically. Keep the additional sheets that follow to update your working heart rate zone or help friends/family calculate theirs.

Use one, or better yet two, of these methods to monitor your heart rate. It's important. One of the biggest reasons why people detest exercise is because they think it will be too difficult. This couldn't be further from the truth. When you are working out at the level that is right for you, you will feel like you can do it. You will feel capable. Confident. And enjoy how refreshed you are afterwards. You will not feel like you are going to die! That only means you are overdoing it

KARVONEAN FORMULA

Finding your working heart rate and heart rate zone.

Maximal heart rate   220

Subtract your age today   -
                                                      _____

Your resting heart rate
(taken for 1 minute)   -
                                                      _____

Multiply by intensity level   _____   _____
(.60 is lower, .85 is higher)   x   .60   x   .85
                                                _____   _____

Add back resting heart rate   +   +
                                                _____   _____

These 2 numbers represent your
target heart rate range. You
need to workout somewhere in
between. Start at the low end.

Divide by 6. This is what you   =   =
will use in a 10 second count.   _____   _____
From now on you won't have to count
per minute, just 10 seconds.

TARGET HEART RATE RANGE = _____ to_____

KARVONEAN FORMULA EXAMPLE

Finding your working heart rate and heart rate zone

Maximal heart rate	220	
Subtract your age today	- **45**	
	_175_	
Your resting heart rate (taken for 1 minute)	- **65**	
	_110_	_110_
Multiply by intensity level (.60 is lower, .85 is higher)	x .60	x .85
	_66_	_94_
Add back resting heart rate	+ 65	+ 65
These 2 numbers represent your target heart rate range. You need to workout somewhere in between. Start at the low end.	_131_ to	_159_
Divide by 6. This is what you will use in a 10 second count. From now on you won't have to count per minute, just 10 seconds.	_22_ to	_27_

TARGET HEART RATE RANGE = 22 – 27 when using a 10 second count

CHAPTER REFLECTION

Date: _____

What did I learn from this chapter?

What will I do differently or apply this week?

How do I feel after completing this chapter?

HOW MUCH, HOW HARD, HOW LONG?

Just how many days a week, how hard, and how long should you exercise? It all depends upon what you're trying to accomplish. If you simply want to become more active than you already are, several days a week may suffice. However, if you want to lose weight, get your heart and lungs in better shape, increase flexibility, and boost your strength and endurance (in other words, improve your overall health), you'll need to work out at least three times a week.

When you're just starting out, don't push yourself too hard. Work at the difficulty level that is right for you - whatever that may be. Intensity will naturally increase as you get in better and better shape. Always do as much as you feel you can do comfortably. Over time, you naturally will be working harder to get to that point. Your muscles will need more intense movements and activities to achieve the same level of effort. That's called a "training effect," and it just means that you need to elevate your heart rate to a certain level to really get the full benefits out of the exercise.

You already know precisely what your training rate should be, you calculated it in the last chapter. So, that's your guide to "how hard" to exercise.

What if you never quite seem to get your heart rate to where it's supposed to be? There are ways to increase/decrease the intensity or difficulty of your movement. First, the workout will get harder if you increase the range of motion (how far you reach and extend your limbs while performing the activity). If you're walking, for example, you could make the activity harder by using a longer stride (reaching out further with the legs) and using more arm movements. If you find yourself working too hard, the same walk could be made easier by using shorter steps and no arm movements.

Another example would be adding hills to make the exercise harder. As a general rule, to increase difficulty, use more of your legs and arms; to decrease difficulty, use them less. Covering a longer distance or area of space also makes the workout harder whereas a short distance or small area of space will make it easier. For example, exercising in your living room to a video will limit your ability to travel around a large amount of space for harder work.

For how long you should exercise, start with shorter sessions, like 30-40 minutes, and gradually work up to at least an hour. Within that hour you should be able to adequately warm up, work your heart/lungs through aerobic activity, do muscular strength work and end with stretching.

If you feel 20 minutes of activity too challenging, start with less. This is particularly important if you are carrying a lot of extra weight or are less fit. Remember though to go easy. Your muscles, tendons, and ligaments are not used to lifting additional weight so start with only the smallest amount. Most people overestimate their fitness level. Keep in mind that if you do too much too soon you could hinder your training. More importantly, get injured and not be able to exercise at all.

Simply put, exercise at least three times a week, within your target heart rate range, for a minimum of a half hour working up to an hour. Use the work sheet at the end of the chapter to log how much, how hard and how long you are going to begin with.

Writing in which days and times of the week you plan on exercising will assure that you actually have a place in your mind and calendar for an activity program. Make sure to pick times and days that will work on a regular basis. For example, if you work 9 - 5 and frequently stay late, don't pick 5:30 p.m. for your exercise time. If you know you have a therapy appointment every other Tuesday don't pick Tuesdays either. Chances are your schedule won't perfectly fit your new routine but make the best choices available to you. Also, if your schedule fluctuates, pick alternative days/times NOW. Then, when you go through a change it will be easier to go right to plan B without a lapse in your routine.

Will your schedule always work as you have it planned? Absolutely not. Things are bound to come up. Whether it's family, work, friends, people trying to derail you, the list is long. But, if you really choose days and times that have a low probability of getting interfered with you have a much better chance of staying on track.

If you do miss a workout it's not the end of the world. It's not the one workout you miss that's important; it's all the ones that you complete that make a big difference to your health and well-being. Just remember it takes many days to form a new habit. If you want your exercise routine to become a normal part of your life, like brushing your teeth, you'll need to do it regularly enough to make that happen.

HOW MUCH, HOW HARD, HOW LONG WORKSHEET

HOW MUCH?

1. I need to aim for a minimum of three workouts per week.

Plan A will be done on the following days:

_____

And, at the following times:_____

Plan B (my alternate plan in case I need to miss a day/time) will be done on the following days:

_____

And, at the following times:_____

HOW HARD?

Plug in your target heart rate range calculated in the last chapter. Take your heart rate after each aerobic segment and make sure it falls within this range.

_____

HOW LONG?

How long will I exercise during the first week? (This is per exercise session)

_____

CHAPTER REFLECTION

Date: _____

What did I learn from this chapter?

What will I do differently or apply this week?

How do I feel after completing this chapter?

COMMON EXERCISE MYTHS

There are many myths and misconceptions concerning weight loss. It's not surprising if you've gotten discouraged or overwhelmed about getting fit before. Our human desire to see quick results often interferes with basic logic. Even after reading this section, you may find yourself sliding back into erroneous beliefs.

Let's see how much you actually know about exercise and weight loss. Be honest and answer the following questions. Then, rate yourself on the scale that follows. Each question will be discussed later.

True or False:

_____ Fat cells can be eliminated by proper exercise and a good diet.

_____ Sit-ups are good for removing fat from the abdominal area.

_____ In the long run, diet and exercise are equally important in keeping off lost weight.

_____ If you are naturally thin, you don't need to exercise as much as someone who is overweight.

_____ Muscle built up through a weight training program will turn to fat once you stop.

_____ Your scale can accurately tell you how much fat you've lost.

_____ Low-calorie diets lead to a large initial loss of fat.

_____ To sustain itself, a fat cell needs to burn more energy than a muscle cell.

_____ In order to reap benefits from an exercise program you must do at least 30 minutes of strenuous aerobic exercise a minimum of three times per week.

_____ The harder you work out the more fat you burn.

_____ Fat will burn off the body in areas it is most abundant in first.

_____ Losing and gaining weight repeatedly has no effect on future weight loss attempts.

_____ Drinking the right amount of water has no effect on fat loss.

_____ Playing sports, doing gardening, yard work, housework and chasing after kids all day can all keep you in good shape.

_____ Men are not as coordinated as women.

_____ In order for exercise to have done any good, you should experience some soreness the next day.

_____ The adage "No pain, no gain" still holds true - if you don't exercise through the burn you won't get good results.

_____ It takes at least six weeks to reap any benefits from an exercise program.

_____ If women use weight equipment they'll bulk up and look masculine.

_____ As a normal part of aging, there will come a time when it's just too late to exercise.

_____ How many calories an activity burns is important in choosing your form of exercise.

_____ For the obese, water aerobics is the best way to burn fat.

_____ Being overweight and overfat are the same thing.

---- Thigh cream, miracle pills and revolutionary diets advertised in the newspaper and magazines must work otherwise they couldn't be sold.

----- When at the gym, it's a good idea to copy what exercises you see the other members do. Especially if you are new and don't really know how to use the equipment.

_____ Certain foods like celery and cucumber require more energy for digestion, absorption, and metabolism than the calories they provide.

Scoring:

All answers are false. Count up the number of questions you answered "true" to. Do the same for all "false" answers. The more "true" answers you got, the more you need to educate yourself about weight loss and fitness. If you missed just a few, consider yourself way above the average person in terms of fitness knowledge. Correctly answering about half shows you're on the right track but still have enough misconceptions to botch a good routine. On the other hand, if you answered most wrong, don't get down on yourself. These myths are still floating around society and crop up in daily conversations. By just repeating and believing what you hear in passing, you're likely to have answered "true" to most of the above. Now you know what the answers are. Let's find out the "whys" behind each one.

1. Fat cells can be eliminated by proper exercise and a good diet.

No amount of exercise and diet can remove a single fat cell. Unfortunately, fat cells cannot disappear, only shrink or increase in size.

The only way to actually remove fat cells is through surgery such as liposuction, a procedure I do not recommend for anyone unless it is medically imperative and weight loss by other means is impossible.

2. Sit-ups are good for removing fat from the abdominal area.

Sit-ups, push-ups, lunges, and other calisthenics or so-called "toning" exercises will not burn any fat. Traditional spot toning exercises are anaerobic movements and don't take energy from stored fat. In order for any activity to be a fatburning one, it must be aerobic. That is, utilizing the large muscles in the legs continuously to elevate the heart into a training zone for at least 20 minutes in duration. Sit-ups will strengthen and define the abdominal muscles. But unless you burn off the layer of fat on top, you'll never be able to see them. Still perform sit-ups, they're a good exercise for abdominal and back strength - just don't expect them to get rid of a pot belly.

3. In the long run, diet and exercise are equally important in keeping off lost weight.

The consensus still remains that those who continue exercising keep weight off for a longer period of time than those who try to maintain weight through diet alone. With all the benefits of exercise it only makes sense to address both areas.

4. If you are naturally thin, you don't need to exercise as much as someone who is overweight.

Being thin is not necessarily an indicator of good health. A thin person may be more unhealthy than someone a few pounds over their ideal weight. When talking about total health we have to consider how sound the body functions. Are the heart and blood vessels strong? How about the respiratory system? Is the person flexible and do they have a good deal of muscular strength? The person who is thin may be carrying around a larger percentage of body fat than a larger, more fit person. Excess body fat has been associated with strokes, hypertension, arteriosclerosis, varicose veins, respiratory ailments, arthritis, back pain, joint problems, cancer, diabetes, gall bladder diseases, earlier deaths and higher mortality rates in general.

5. Muscle built up through a weight training program will turn to fat once you stop.

You can't turn muscle into fat any more than you can turn an apple into an orange. Muscle cells and fat cells are separate entities. When fat is burned off and muscle mass increased, the appearance of the body becomes lean and defined. If exercise is removed at that point, the body just slowly reverts back to its pre-exercise state. Once again, fat accumulates over the muscles and without toning exercises, muscles atrophy. You simply have smaller muscles and more body fat.

6. Your scale can accurately tell you how much fat you've lost.

Your scale can never, ever, ever, ever, tell you how much fat you've lost! The only information a scale can accurately reflect is how much you weigh. That weight can be any combination of fat, muscle, water and more. In my opinion, stepping on and off a scale sets you up for eventual disappointment and depression. It's very possible to be on a successful weight loss program and not show a loss on the scale. How can that be? Well, muscle weighs more than an equal amount of fat. If you burn off fat and replace it with more muscle you may not see any pound loss. It's even possible to see a gain. At least when first starting out. Think about some of the athletes you see on TV. Tennis players, skiers, skaters, etc. Any one of them weigh a lot more than an average person of the same height. Muscle is why. The scale can also fool you into thinking you are losing fat when indeed you've only dehydrated yourself or lost valuable muscle. To accurately measure your fat loss you must choose a more precise measurement - like using a tape measure or body fat analysis.

7. Low-calorie diets lead to a large initial loss of fat.

Low-calorie diets lead to a loss of pounds on the scale but don't necessarily initiate fat loss. Any diet lower than 1000-1200 calories a day may be dangerous. Losing more than 1-2 pounds a week most likely means you're losing other things besides fat. What usually happens when you go on a very low-calorie diet is that water, electrolytes, some fat and even muscle is broken down and excreted from the body. This shows up as a great weight loss. Then, after a few days, the body acclimates to the lower intake of calories and starts slowing down it's metabolic rate to survive comfortably on less fuel. You then burn calories at a slower rate and show smaller weight losses on the scale. Extremely low-calorie diets are usually done under the supervision of a medical doctor for a reason - they can be very dangerous.

8. To sustain itself, a fat cell needs to burn more energy than a muscle cell.

Even at rest, a given number of muscle cells will be utilizing more energy and burning more calories than the same number of fat cells. The nice thing about being fit and having more muscle is that your body will be using more calories all around thereby increasing your metabolism. Fat cells require much less energy to keep themselves nourished and alive. So, if you're going to weigh 140 lbs., aim to make that 140 lbs. more muscle than fat.

9. In order to reap benefits from an exercise program you must do at least 30 minutes of strenuous aerobic exercise a minimal of three times per week.

The ACSM (American College of Sports Medicine) is now stating that every minute of exercise is beneficial no matter when and where it is done. Certainly, you need aerobic exercise to help with fat burning and cardiovascular health but if the only other alternative is being sedentary, do something. Anything will be better than complete inactivity.

10. The harder you work out the more fat you burn.

Fat burns at a moderate, not high, intensity. That means when you push yourself to the point where you can't breathe comfortably or feel burning muscles you're not working at an aerobic pace. Working out at extremely high levels may be fine for conditioned athletes but the average person receives no benefit by doing so.

For the best results, when it comes to fat loss, the important thing is duration or how long you perform the activity. Working at a moderate difficulty for a longer period of time will give you greater results and slowly condition you for harder work if and when you choose to do it.

11. Fat will burn off the body in areas it is most abundant in first.

Many times people ask how to get fat off a particular body area. Unfortunately, there is no secret. Fat will burn off all areas of the body and many times it comes off the most abundant areas last. Focusing on the back of your arm or your stomach won't help you remove fat any faster. Consistent aerobic exercise is the only way. Over time, it will come off.

12. Losing and gaining weight repeatedly has no effect on future weight loss attempts.

Studies have shown that repeated weight loss and gain makes it much more likely that future attempts at weight loss will fail. In addition, studies also point out a relationship between earlier deaths and yo-yo dieting. If you are planning on embarking on a quick weight loss cure, don't. You're safer not doing anything than having your weight fluctuate up and down over and over again. Find a sensible approach, something you can live with and take it one day at a time.

13. Drinking the right amount of water has no effect on fat loss.

Water is necessary for breaking down fat. The liver breaks down stored fat for energy. The kidneys need water for excretion. When you don't drink enough water, the kidneys can't work to their capacity and force some of their work onto the liver. As a result, the liver metabolizes less fat and you don't lose weight. The larger the person, the greater the need for water. Water also works to suppress the appetite, alleviate constipation, flush out waste and prevent dehydration. Don't underestimate the role of water in a weight loss program. Drink at least 8 glasses a day (including juices, sodas, coffee, etc.).

14. Playing golf, doing gardening, yard work, housework and chasing after kids all day can all keep you in good shape.

Although certain sports can keep you fit if they are strenuous and continuous enough, as a general rule games like golf, and all the other above activities cannot keep you in good all-around shape. As mentioned before, you need aerobic activity for at least 20 minutes at a time to ensure fat burning and cardiovascular conditioning. Stop and go activities such as the above don't fit that category and can't give you all of the many benefits of a structured fitness program.

15. Men are not as coordinated as women.

Men may feel less coordinated than women but aren't. Women grow up partaking in activities that involve body awareness and movement much more so than men. Usually the only experience men can fall back on is their athletic skills. The key to coordination is practice. Whether it's country line dancing or pickleball, you have to get enough practice to become accomplished with the steps and getting your body to move the way you want it to.

16. In order for exercise to have done any good, you should experience some soreness the next day.

Getting sore is not a good sign. In fact, it's a message to you that you've done more than your body is ready to do. I've heard many times the comment "I got sore but that's good! It means I did something." Unless you're the Marquis de Sade, post-exercise pain is not pleasurable. Aim to feel your muscles working during the workout, not locked up the next day. Slight tightness in the muscles is something else. Usually, when you've done the right amount of exercise, you'll feel tighter the next day but not incapacitated.

17. The adage "No pain, no gain" still holds true - if you don't exercise through the burn you won't get good results.

Exercising through a burn is not only uncomfortable, but also counterproductive. The burn is actually a buildup of a waste product in the bloodstream called lactic acid. As lactic acid levels increase, fatigue sets in. When you don't allow lactic acid levels to reach that point you can do more exercises total. Here's an example. Say you are going to do push-ups. You do 10 and you start to feel burning. You keep going and do maybe three more before your muscles completely fatigue. You've done 13 in all. A better way would be to do the same

10 push-ups. At the first sensation of burning, rest for several seconds. Start again until you feel burning. Continue until you have fatigued the muscles. This way you are certain to do more push-ups total and thus increase your strength and endurance much quicker.

18. It takes at least six weeks to reap any benefits from an exercise program.

Absolutely not! Observable improvements are often not seen for four to six weeks but gains in strength, flexibility, coordination and endurance are achieved much sooner. Psychological aspects such as improved mood, increased self-esteem and stress reduction are apparent after the very first session. Biological benefits such as sleeping better, more energy and decreased appetite are also seen immediately. Six weeks is usually mentioned as the time needed to see results but keep in mind that's only the visible ones.

19. If women use weight equipment they'll bulk up and look masculine.

Women don't have the amount of male hormone (testosterone) necessary for bulking up. No matter how hard they work, how often or how much weight they use they'll never have the bulky looking muscles of a man. In the past, women bodybuilders have taken steroids which allow them to develop muscles larger than they could ever do on their own. These are the women who look masculine, large and unattractive. Look at the women bodybuilders today - they aren't hulks; they just have wonderful, sculpted muscles and don't have much fat on their bodies. With so much of the focus on "aerobic" exercise for fat loss, "anaerobic" exercise such as weight training is often overlooked. The weights can give you more shape, definition and a more sculpted look than aerobic exercise alone can produce.

20. As a normal part of aging, there will come a time when it's too late to exercise.

You'll never be too old to exercise. You can improve your general health and the quality of life no matter when you begin to move. Normal aging may prevent you from performing some of the movements you could do years ago. That doesn't mean you can't find other suitable alternatives. There are thousands of activities and movements to choose from. Even simple walking or exercises done in a wheelchair can greatly improve your health. Jack Lalanne swam and lifted weights until the day he died, at 96. It's never too late!

21. How many calories an activity burns is important in choosing your form of exercise.

Who cares how many calories the activity burns if it's not something you enjoy enough to do regularly? The first and foremost consideration in choosing your form of exercise is picking something you like. Is it enjoyable to you? Will you do it enough to get any results? Don't go any further until you've come up with something to fit the description of "fun".

22. For the obese, water aerobics is the best way to burn fat.

Experts disagree as to whether or not water aerobics programs effectively burn fat. The temperature of the water is one factor. The colder the water, the more likely fat reserves will remain to keep the body warm. Why should the body shed fat when it needs it to keep it warm? Also, body fat increases buoyancy making it easier to float and move through the water. In general, having more body fat in water is a biological advantage if you think about ease of movement and heat insulation. On the other hand, you are burning a substantial amount of calories in the water. By controlling your diet, those calories are going to have to come from somewhere. Most likely from fat. If you love water aerobics classes, don't give them up. Add other aerobic activities to your routine though, such as walking or biking.

23. Being overweight and overfat are the same thing.

Someone can be overweight but not be overfat. Overweight refers to what is generally acceptable as the weight you should be at. Height and weight charts give a range of what weight is acceptable for your height. Overfat refers to the internal composition of your body. In other words, a measure of what percentage of fat you have in relation to muscle and water. Maybe you weigh exactly what you are supposed to according to a height/weight chart. You can still be overfat. In fact, no matter how thin you are, you can still be overfat. When the percentage of fat within the body exceeds a given number (the upper limit for general health is 25%-31% for women, 18%-24% for men), you are overfat and more susceptible to illness and certain diseases.

24. Thigh cream, miracle pills and revolutionary diets advertised in the news and magazines must work otherwise they couldn't be sold.

Positively no. No amount of cream or concoction of herbs is going to burn any fat. Promoters are able to advertise their products provided there is always a recommendation for the user to eat a sensible diet and exercise regularly. Anyone who eats a sensible diet and exercises regularly is going to lose weight - with or without some magic pill they happen to be taking at the same time. If you don't believe it try it yourself. Buy a package of m & m's or saltine crackers. Re-package them and either get two friends to take part or do it yourself. Eat one cracker or m & m at each meal. Make sure you eat a low fat diet and don't go over 1200 calories a day. Also make sure you exercise 30 minutes every day. At the end of the month, you or your friends will most likely have lost weight. But not from the "miracle cure" you gave them - only by being bluffed into doing what is needed to lose weight effectively anyway. These scam artists are conning you. I guess they feel justified that they're selling you something that can get you to eat good and work out. Unfortunately though, the exercise and diet recommendations get chucked into the trash. People try to get the product to do the work instead of themselves and of course it doesn't. Start looking at the advertisements on weight loss products. You will see, in small print usually at the bottom of the page, the reference to diet and exercise.

25. When at the gym, it's a good idea to copy what exercises you see the other members do. Especially if you are new and don't really know how to use the equipment.

Absolutely not! This is something that is very common in fitness facilities. Each person in there is doing something that is at their level. Their level is not yours. In addition, there is no guarantee that what they are doing is even safe. Copying what someone else is doing can be one of the most dangerous things you can do in a club setting. A lot of times I see this with stretching. People are doing stretches that they did 30 years ago and are no longer considered safe or effective. They are setting themselves up for injuries and leading others towards risk by their example.

26. Certain foods like celery and cucumber require more energy for digestion, absorption, and metabolism than the calories they provide.

No. The concept that there are negative calorie foods has never had any science behind it.

BOGUS FITNESS DEVICES

Everywhere you turn there seems to be someone touting the benefits of a new fitness device or trend. The claims are exciting and lure people into spending a lot of money that does little or nothing to help with overall fitness. Here are some examples of products to stay away from. Although they may make your body feel good, they don't have any solid studies backing significant weight loss or fitness enhancing claims.

Vibration Platforms: The claim is that users burn calories and improve muscle tone by standing or exercising on a vibrating platform. While they can provide a sense of muscle engagement, the overall health benefits and weight loss claims have been met with skepticism. More studies need to be done to determine if there are indeed benefits.

Electric Muscle Stimulation (EMS) Devices for Weight Loss: There are gadgets that claim to help users lose weight by sending electrical impulses to stimulate muscles. While EMS can be beneficial for rehabilitation and certain fitness purposes, its effectiveness for weight loss is debated, and relying solely on such devices without a proper diet and exercise plan may not yield significant results.

Passive Exercise Machines: Devices that claim to mimic the effects of exercise without the need for physical exertion have been criticized. For example, gadgets that claim to provide the benefits of cardiovascular exercise without actually moving the body extensively may not be as effective as traditional forms of exercise.

Slimming Belts and Sauna Suits: Products that claim to help users lose weight by promoting sweating, such as sauna suits or slimming belts, are often criticized for providing temporary water weight loss rather than actual fat loss. The weight lost through sweating is quickly regained once the user rehydrates.

Ab Stimulators and Toning Belts: Devices that claim to tone and strengthen abdominal muscles through electrical stimulation have been met with skepticism regarding their effectiveness for achieving visible results comparable to traditional core exercises.

Hula Hoops with Added Weight or Vibrations: While traditional hula hooping can be a fun and effective form of exercise, some versions of weighted or vibrating hula hoops claim to enhance calorie burn and slim the waist. The efficacy of these variations has been debated.

Gravity Boots: These boots are designed for hanging upside down to decompress the spine. While inversion therapy has its merits for certain back issues, the use of gravity boots for general fitness or weight loss has not been validated.

Treadmill Workstations or Under-Desk Exercise Machines: While the idea of staying active while working is commendable, some under-desk exercise machines or treadmill workstations may not provide a sufficient workout to replace dedicated exercise sessions. The ability to effectively multitask while using these devices is also debated.

Resistance Band Shoes: Shoes with built-in resistance bands claim to provide extra resistance during daily activities, with the goal of toning leg muscles. The effectiveness of these shoes for achieving meaningful muscle engagement is uncertain.

Isometric Exercise Devices: Isometric exercise involves static muscle contractions without joint movement. In other words, you tighten or hold your muscles in one position without moving the joint. Some gadgets claim to provide isometric workouts for various muscle groups. The effectiveness of these devices may be limited compared to dynamic resistance exercises.

Breathing Exercise Devices: Devices designed to train and strengthen respiratory muscles for improved lung capacity and breathing. While beneficial for specific health conditions, their effectiveness for general fitness may be limited compared to traditional cardiovascular exercises.

Posture Correction Gadgets: Wearable devices that claim to improve posture through reminders or gentle vibrations. While maintaining good posture is crucial for overall health, the effectiveness of these gadgets in achieving lasting posture improvements is debated.

Body Vibration Massagers: These devices use vibrations to target muscles for massage and relaxation. While they can provide relief for sore muscles, their ability to replace traditional massages or contribute significantly to fitness is a subject of discussion

Hand Grip Strength Trainers: Devices designed to strengthen hand and forearm muscles by providing resistance during squeezing. While these gadgets can be useful for specific goals, their overall impact on general fitness is limited compared to comprehensive strength training.

Jump Training Shoes: Shoes with built-in platforms or springs that claim to enhance vertical jump height and overall athletic performance. The effectiveness and safety of these shoes for long-term use are areas of debate.

FAD DIETS

We tend to attach two meanings to the word "diet," so it gets confusing. Are we talking about an eating style? Or are we talking about a list of specific foods we're going to be eating for a specified period of time? In this section I'm going to be talking about highly restrictive diets. Fad diets.

Fad diets are popular, often temporary eating plans that promise quick weight loss or other health benefits, but they are typically not supported by long-term scientific evidence. Many times these diets come with celebrity endorsements which make them super appealing. Still, diets that focus on a few food items are not good for your overall health. They eliminate all the healthy foods that you need for a healthy body and mind. Often, they can lead to nutrient deficiencies or health issues. They also are not sustainable, which means at some point you will go off them. When that happens you're back to square one and will resume eating what you did before. They may in fact lead to more harm than good. Here are some examples:

Keto Diet: High-fat, low-carb diet that puts the body into ketosis, where fat is burned for energy instead of carbohydrates. For anyone with kidney disease, liver conditions, pancreatitis, diabetes or heart disease it can be dangerous.

Paleo Diet: Focuses on eating foods thought to be available to early humans, such as meat, fish, fruits, and vegetables, while avoiding processed foods, grains, and dairy.

Atkins Diet: Another low-carb diet that allows high amounts of protein and fat, limiting carbohydrates to encourage weight loss.

Juice Cleanses: Involves consuming only fruit and vegetable juices for several days to "detox" the body, often resulting in quick weight loss but lacking essential nutrients.

Cabbage Soup Diet: Centers on eating cabbage soup multiple times a day along with small amounts of other low-calorie foods for rapid weight loss.

Raw Food Diet: Advocates consuming uncooked, unprocessed foods, usually plant-based, to preserve nutrients and enzymes.

Master Cleanse: A liquid diet consisting of lemon juice, maple syrup, cayenne pepper, and water, claimed to detox the body and promote weight loss.

HCG Diet: Combines extreme calorie restriction (500 calories per day) with HCG hormone supplements, which is highly controversial and unsafe.

South Beach Diet: Focuses on reducing carbs and increasing protein and healthy fats in phases to stabilize blood sugar levels and promote weight loss.

Alkaline Diet: Encourages eating foods that make the body more alkaline (fruits, vegetables, nuts) and avoiding acidic foods (meat, dairy, processed foods), though the body regulates pH naturally.

Blood Type Diet: Proposes that people should eat according to their blood type (A, B, AB, O), with specific foods recommended for each type to improve health and digestion. There is little scientific evidence to support this theory.

Zone Diet: Encourages eating a specific ratio of macronutrients (40% carbs, 30% protein, 30% fat) at every meal to control insulin levels and promote weight loss and energy balance.

5:2 Diet: A form of intermittent fasting where you eat normally for five days a week and drastically reduce calorie intake (500-600 calories) for two days.

The Grapefruit Diet: A low-calorie diet that includes eating grapefruit or drinking grapefruit juice with every meal, believed to help burn fat. There is no strong evidence supporting this.

The Beverly Hills Diet: Focuses on the idea that fruit contains enzymes that help burn fat. For the first 10 days, only fruit is allowed, followed by gradual introduction of carbs and proteins.

The Military Diet: A very low-calorie diet that claims to help you lose 10 pounds in a week by following a strict meal plan for three days, followed by four days of normal eating.

SlimFast Diet: Replaces two meals a day with meal replacement shakes and encourages a third "sensible" meal. It's marketed for quick weight loss, but it's not a sustainable long-term solution for many.

Raw Till 4: A vegan diet that promotes eating raw fruits and vegetables until 4 PM, then eating a cooked, plant-based meal for dinner. Critics argue it may lack sufficient nutrients, especially protein.

The Baby Food Diet: Involves replacing meals or snacks with jars of baby food to cut calories and control portion sizes. This lacks variety and doesn't offer the nutrients needed for adult health.

Dukan Diet: A high-protein, low-carb diet in four phases, starting with mainly lean protein and eventually adding vegetables, carbs, and fats. It promotes rapid weight loss but can be restrictive and difficult to maintain.

Cotton Ball Diet: An extreme and dangerous fad where individuals eat cotton balls dipped in juice or other liquids to suppress appetite. This can lead to serious digestive issues and malnutrition.

Tapeworm Diet: This bizarre and hazardous practice involves ingesting a tapeworm to "eat" excess calories. It is illegal, unsafe, and can lead to serious health problems.

The Ice Diet: Suggests eating ice to burn calories, based on the idea that the body uses energy to heat the ice. This approach lacks substantial evidence and would likely result in minimal weight loss.

Breatharian Diet: A highly dangerous and pseudoscientific belief that people can survive on just sunlight and air without food or water. This has been linked to severe malnutrition and death.

Yes, the above have all been promoted as a great way to lose weight but if you really want to go on a legitimate, effective weight loss diet, go for a Mediterranean or Plant-Based one for optimal health benefits. Those diets are backed up by numerous studies and wellness experts.

These are just some of the many myths you come across daily. Remind yourself to find out how much (or little) truth is in what you hear, especially before you repeat it to someone else. If you're not sure, check with credible sources like The Nutrition Source from Harvard's School of Public Health or The American College of Sports Medicine (ACSM).

Believing misinformation can destroy the most successful fitness or weight management program in the world. Before you even get started! There's no quick fix to getting in shape or changing what you look like. Just like with other goals you achieve, there's no magic involved. It takes time, patience and determination. Now that you know what doesn't work, it's time to dive into what does…

CHAPTER REFLECTION

Date: _____

What did I learn from this chapter?

What will I do differently or apply this week?

How do I feel after completing this chapter?

YOUR CUSTOMIZED FITNESS PLAN

Now it's time to design your plan! A plan that WILL work because it is tailored to fit your personality, needs and goals. It will require thought, so be sure to take time to think through this section. It's very important to create the ideal plan that will work for you. This way you'll be motivated to do it and it will endure over time. And most importantly, it will provide you the results you want.

The next pages have a worksheet that will help you create your customized plan. As time goes on, the plan may need to be adjusted. Particularly once it gets too easy for you or you see a recurring stumbling block. That's to be expected. But for now, tap into what you've already learned about your fears, feelings, mindset and motivational style so that your mental foundation gets worked into your plan. Will it be perfect? No. Will it help you learn more about yourself so that you can refine it and keep moving forward? Yes!

SETTING GOALS

Most of us don't get in our cars and just start driving. We usually have a destination in mind. Taking the time to think about and set goals is one of the most important things you can do to ensure the success of your fitness program. What is it that you actually want to accomplish? Do you know? Perhaps it's getting your doctor to stop reprimanding you. Or maybe you hope to reduce stress, get rid of fatigue or sleep better. Possibly your goals are more like losing 20 pounds, walking up a flight of stairs without getting winded or reducing pain from a chronic illness like arthritis or diabetes. Whatever the reason, it's important you write down what your individual goals are. It helps keep you focused on what you want to achieve.

When crafting your goals, be realistic. It's not realistic to expect yourself to drive nonstop from one side of the country to another, any more than you can expect to drop 50 lbs. in a month. Realistic goals function to help you stay on track.

A good way to set realistic goals is to use the SMART approach. SMART meaning Specific, Measurable, Achievable, Relevant, and Time-bound.

Here's an example: John joined a local fitness boot camp with the goal of losing weight and building strength. Initially, his goal was vague, and he grew discouraged by how much heavier the weights felt to him compared to others in the class. After struggling to complete sets and constantly comparing himself to his peers, John began doubting his ability to succeed.

However, after a conversation with a supportive instructor, he decided to apply a more structured approach by setting a SMART goal. He refined his goal to be more specific, focusing on improving his strength and health at his own pace. He decided to attend boot camp three times a week and track his progress by noting the weights he lifted, the number of sets he completed, and how often he showed up to class.

To make his goal measurable, John aimed to increase his weights by 5% every two weeks and add an extra set whenever possible. Recognizing the importance of keeping his goal achievable, he committed to focusing on his personal growth rather than comparing himself to others. That meant making small, steady improvements without overwhelming himself. His goal was also relevant to his overall desire to lead a healthier lifestyle, which had always been a priority for him. Finally, John set a time-bound target: in three months, he wanted to lift 10% more weight than when he started and maintain consistent attendance at boot camp.

With this SMART approach, John shifted his mindset from comparison to self-improvement. He began to celebrate small victories, like completing an extra set or increasing his weights slightly and found greater satisfaction in his workouts. Over time, he no longer felt defeated by his peers' progress and instead appreciated his own journey. By keeping his goals clear, measurable, and focused on his own abilities, John saw significant improvements in both his strength and overall fitness.

YOUR GOALS

Here are some examples of goals. You may have very different ones. What matters is that you write them down. They help give you a clear vision of what you hope to achieve through this fitness journey. Whenever you feel discouraged, revisit the list to remind yourself of the personal reasons driving your commitment to exercise.

- **Improve Health**: "I will lower my blood pressure by 10 points and reduce my risk of diabetes within the next 6 months."

- **Increase Energy**: "I will increase my energy levels over the next year so that I can play with my kids for 30 minutes after work, three times a week, without feeling exhausted."

- **Boost Confidence**: "I will fit into a size 14 within six months."

- **Social Engagement**: "I will share my fitness progress on social media once a week for the next three months to engage with friends and family and receive their support."

Be careful when writing down goals for weight loss. Keep in mind that under the best circumstances (eating right and exercising daily) losing 1-2 pounds per week is considered safe, gradual weight loss. True weight loss means losing fat slowly enough that you are more likely to keep it off.

Think of body fat like a bank account where you store extra energy (calories). When you eat more calories than your body needs, it stores the extra energy as fat. It takes 3,500 extra calories to store one pound of fat in your body.

So, to lose one pound of fat, you need to "burn off" 3,500 calories. This doesn't mean you have to burn all those calories in one day—it can be done gradually. For example, if you reduce your daily calorie intake by 500 calories (or burn 500 calories through exercise), you'll create a deficit of 3,500 calories over the course of a week, resulting in about one pound of fat loss.

I like to look at it as if calories are money. Each day I have 2200 of them to use as I wish. But, once they're used up, I'm done eating for the day. This allows one to be very conscious of different calorie values of foods and different food choices. Would you rather have a large healthy salad for dinner or a small order of French fries from a fast food establishment? It's your choice.

Once you get familiar with how many calories are in the foods you eat, you'll naturally start making better food choices. Go back to the Food Ledger you filled out from Chapter 6 and add up the number of calories you typically eat in one day. Then you can strive to eat 500 less. If you're not sure how to do that and are hesitant to make any major changes to your eating habits up front, just start eating less. Cut your portions in half and you'll start the fat burning process without making big changes in your food selection.

For now, fill out the following fitness plan so you can start designing and refining your program.

FITNESS PLAN WORKSHEET

A. Top Goals

Write down your 3 most important goals. Choose goals that are SMART.

_____

_____

_____

Which forms of exercise would help you achieve those goals (Use the Exercise Selection Guide in the previous chapter and list any/all that you think could help you achieve your goals.).

_____

_____

_____

B. Restrictions?

What are your restrictions? Refine your suggested choices above in order to work around your limitations.

_____

_____

_____

C. Fun

List eight activities from the previous chapter's list of suggestions that you would most enjoy doing regularly (or hate the least). You can see yourself doing these things, even if a bit awkward or uncomfortable at first. Pick two from each of the categories that cover the components of fitness. That means include aerobic exercise, strength, endurance and flexibility

1.

2.

3.

4.

5.

6.

7.

8.

D. Motivation

List 2 ways to make each of the above activities externally motivating (involving other people):

1.   and

2.   and

3.   and

4.   and

5.   and

6.   and

7.   and

8.   and

F. Which activities do you think you will enjoy the most? Why? Come back after a month of dong your plan and see if you were right.

_____

_____

CHAPTER REFLECTION

Date: _____

What did I learn from this chapter?

What will I do differently or apply this week?

How do I feel after completing this chapter?

RECORDING YOUR PROGRESS

If you decide to go for a 100-mile drive, you won't know how far you've gone without knowing what the odometer read when you started. The same concept is true when it comes to getting fit. How can you possibly know you've improved unless you know where you were when you started? Using the mirror or the scale to tell you about improvement is not the best way to go. For one thing, the more body fat you have, the less likely you'll see visual fat loss the first month or so in the mirror. If you judge your progress solely by what you see in the mirror, you may feel like you're not making any headway when in fact you may be doing great. Many internal benefits are occurring long before any changes are visible to the eye. And scales are misleading. The number you see when you step on the scale does not tell you how many pounds of fat you have nor whether you've just lost a pound of fat or a pound of water. I've known people who gave up a terrific exercise program because they didn't *feel* like they were getting anything out of it. Don't let this happen to you!

Chart your improvements from day one onward. Use the following Progress Sheet as your guide. When you test yourself on day one and again six weeks later, you'll definitely see the improvement on paper, much more so than in the mirror.

Keep your progress notes somewhere visible so you can glance at them regularly. They'll help keep you motivated to continue. It's much harder to quit when you know you've lost 5-6 inches and increased your flexibility by an inch than when you're not sure if you've accomplished anything. Give yourself this advantage from the beginning because an exercise program without monitoring is hard to sustain.

In addition to seeing your gains on paper, you'll also be able to key into any problems in your routine. For example, you consistently lose several inches every six week period for four months and then all of a sudden the inch loss stops. You know that events within the last six weeks need to be looked over - maybe you notice your eating has been out of control, you've hit an exercise plateau, need to make minor modifications to your exercise routine (maybe now it's too short, too long, too hard, too easy for where you're at now) or deal with motivational issues.

It's much easier pinpointing problems that stem back six weeks instead of four months. Think about it like monitoring your checking account balance. If you wait four months to identify an error it's a lot more difficult to correct it going through months of transactions than if you caught it right away.

Before you start any exercise, complete the Fitness Test located at the end of the chapter. Make sure you put a date on it and write in the date for re-testing in six weeks. There are other tests available that are much more intensive and you can find them in most physical education or exercise instruction manuals. The one provided here is as brief and basic as possible. You can easily do the assessment in a short amount of time. You also don't need expensive equipment or monitoring devices.

Make sure to replicate the conditions under which you originally tested yourself for all future measurements. Wear the same clothes when you measure. Be aware that uplifting music, proper exercise technique or exercising with others are just a few situations which may allow you to perform optimally.

Poor diet, time of day, medication and numerous other factors could negatively impact your results. You don't need to be a research scientist but keep the above in mind - you don't want to sabotage the numbers in any way if you can help it.

Just tell yourself the numbers will be meaningless the first time. They serve only as a reference point. For our purposes, it doesn't matter what your measurements are on day one or how many sit-ups you can do. The critical issue is whether or not those numbers show an improvement when taken again over time. So, if you're the kind of person who gets depressed when you see your waist size, keep in mind that's where you are today but not where you'll be after settling into a customized fitness routine that is right for you. Focus on improvements only. While you can't change where you are today, you can certainly create a positive change for tomorrow and beyond.

FITNESS TEST INSTRUCTIONS

STRENGTH / ENDURANCE

To test for strength/endurance you'll be doing push-ups, sit-ups and wall sitting. Have a stopwatch or clock with a second hand nearby.

Push-Ups - These can be done in four different ways, according to your own fitness level. If you've never exercised, have a joint, back, weight problem are pregnant or over 50 years old, choose version 1 or 2. If you've been active and fit several other times in your life you can choose version 3 or 4. Just indicate which version you're using so you can repeat the test with the same form.

- Version 1 - Do these standing with your legs 2-3 feet away from a wall. Hands are placed on the wall with arms open wide. Keep hands at chest height, fingers pointing up. Lower and lift your body to and from the wall as if you were a plank. Count each repetition and write down how many you can do without feeling a burn in the muscles.

- Version 2 - On your knees, place hands at shoulder level at a comfortable width. Keeping the back straight bend from the hips and waist using the upper body to absorb the weight as you lower to the ground. This looks like a "girls" push-up except your rear is in the air.

- Version 3 - Similar to the above. Done on the knees but keep back straight as you lower and lift the body to the floor. Find a mirror to perform this to make sure you're doing it properly. Always make sure the back is straight while lowering and lifting. If you see sagging or feel the back pull, do version 2 instead.

- Version 4 - Traditional man's type push up-done on both feet. If you're already quite strong you may want to try this one. For most people though, it will be too difficult if not impossible to do. In order to do the push-up correctly you must keep your entire body tight and straight each time you lift and lower to the ground. Sagging in the back means you're not strong enough to do this yet.

Choose the version you plan on doing and practice a few times, making sure you are comfortable with doing at least a few properly.

Sit-Ups - Lie down on your back with your feet placed firmly on the wall. Your knees should be bent in a right angle and your rear directly underneath your knees. Place both hands behind your head and keep your elbows as open as you can, attempting to keep them away from your view. With your head resting in the hands, slowly lift the chest from the floor towards the ceiling and back down again. Make sure you do this slowly and go to the very highest point you can without jerking your head or pulling on your neck. Practice doing this movement a few times before you actually do the measurement. It takes time to really learn how to relax the neck and head when doing effective sit-ups. Don't expect to be able to lift all the way to your knees either, you'll be doing great if you can get several inches off the floor.

Wall Sit - You need a stopwatch or second hand for this. Stand with your back leaning on a strong wall. Slowly lower your body until you reach a 90 degree angle with your knees. You should appear and feel as if you are in a sitting position. Your back remains against the wall and your feet are directly under your knees. Sit in this position until you begin to feel burning in the leg muscles and can't go on. Stand up and record your time.

FLEXIBILITY

For flexibility you'll need a tape measure or yardstick.

Hamstring - Warm up your muscles by walking around the room half a dozen times and doing some marching in place for a minute or two. Sit with your back to a wall with a yardstick placed against your heels facing away from you. Zero marks where your feet are, all the numbers starting with one are located farther away from you. Reach forward with both hands over the toes. If you can touch the toes, you have a score of "0". If you can reach over your toes, your score is the inch number of how far over you can reach. This is expressed as a plus number such as +1". You may not be able to reach to the toes at all. If this is the case simply turn the yardstick so it faces the other direction and record your number as a negative number, i.e.. - 1 1/2".

Chest - With a tape measure held firmly between the fingers of one hand at the zero point. Hold the middle of the tape loosely in the fingers of the other. Raise both arms overhead. Bring arms behind the head and down behind the back. As you drop the arms the tape measure will slide through the fingers it is held loosely in. When you get to the widest position you are capable of, let go of the firmly held end and write down the number the other fingers are touching.

Adductor - This measures the stretching ability of the inner thigh muscles. Sit upright with feet in front of you and soles of shoes together. Knees will be bent and the outside of the legs will be facing the floor. Press gently down on the legs while keeping feet together. Measure the distance of the kneecap from the floor on each side.

CARDIOVASCULAR ENDURANCE

Cardiovascular endurance is measured using a four inch step and a stopwatch or clock with a second hand.

Resting Heart Rate - This is your heart rate at complete rest. Ideally it should be taken first thing in the morning before you get up and start moving around. Low resting heart rates are associated with higher levels of health and vice versa.

Target Heart Rate Zone - The rate at which your heart should be beating during exercise to give your heart and lungs conditioning benefit and help you burn fat. Use the calculations you arrived at in Chapter 3 for this.

Recovery Heart Rate - How fast your heart is beating shortly after strenuous exercise stops. Your recovery heart rate is a good indicator of how much stronger your heart is getting. As you get in better condition, the heart will bounce back from the strenuous activity faster thus returning to its normal rate of functioning much sooner. Take the pulse at the end of strenuous activity. One minute later take it again, this will be your recovery heart rate.

MEASUREMENTS

Using a tape measure, loosely hold the tape around the fullest part of each body segment. Keep the same tension on the tape every time you measure. If you have someone else measuring you (a friend or co-exerciser) make sure you have the same person re-measure you in six weeks. Each person measures differently and those differences can add up to false results both positive and negative. The areas to be measured are:

- Chest - Under the arms and around the fullest part of bust

- Waist - At the smallest area of the waist

- Hips - At the largest area of the buttocks

- Thighs (L + R) - At the highest point of the thigh

- Knees (L + R) - Just above the knee joint

- Arms (L + R) - Around the fullest part of the upper arm

- Calves (L + R) - At largest part of lower leg

On the next page record your measurements and note the date they were taken (the day you are starting your fitness program). Remeasure in six weeks and again after 12. You will see the progress through gradual inch loss over time.

PROGRESS SHEET

Name_____   Age:_____   Height_____   Weight_____

MEASUREMENTS:

	Date #1:	Date #2:	Date #3:
Chest.............................	_____	_____	_____
Waist.............................	_____	_____	_____
Hips.............................	_____	_____	_____
Thighs (R + L).................	____/___	____/___	____/___
Arms (R + L).................	____/___	____/___	____/___

STRENGTH:

Push-ups.........................	_____	_____	_____
Wall-sit............................	_____	_____	_____
Crunches........................	_____	_____	_____

FLEXIBILITY:

Chest..............................	_____	_____	_____
Hamstring........................	_____	_____	_____
Straddle..........................	_____	_____	_____
Split...............................	_____	_____	_____

CARDIOVASCULAR ENDURANCE:

Resting Heart Rate..........	_____	_____	_____
Recovery Heart Rate.......	_____	_____	_____

BODY COMPOSITION:

	_____	_____	_____

CHAPTER REFLECTION

Date: _____

What did I learn from this chapter?

What will I do differently or apply this week?

How do I feel after completing this chapter?

MY COMMITMENT

You're almost ready to go. Just one more thing. Your personal promise to do your best to fulfill your plan. Make a firm commitment now on the Fitness Contract that follows. Bring in the support of at least one other person. Make sure your support person is truly encouraging of your efforts. It can be anyone you feel will be excited and uplifting to you along the way. The last thing you need is a jealous friend or insecure spouse pretending to be supportive of you when deep down, they *don't* want you to succeed.

If you really don't have a single person you think could be supportive and helpful then fill out the contract by yourself. You'll need more determination and dedication but you can still do it and make it work!

Next, make a commitment as to what you decided on your plan in order to achieve the chosen goals. Write that down as well. Come up with a reward you can give yourself when you actually reach your goal. Make it a tangible perk, something that will serve as a visual reminder that you set a goal and succeeded at making it become a reality. It can be a new outfit, jewelry, a magazine subscription, a new book, a tool, anything that you really would like and are willing to reward yourself with.

It doesn't have to cost money either. Maybe an outing where you take pictures. A day at the beach, in the library or visiting a free museum. Either way, treat yourself to something tangible. Every time you see that reward it will signal to you that you hit a goal. Note this on the Fitness Contract and sign it.

Keep your contract on the refrigerator or somewhere visible where you'll see it every day. It acts like a constant reminder of your commitment, similar to how a runner stays focused when they can see the finish line ahead. When your goal is always in sight, it becomes easier to stay motivated and push through any challenges because you can clearly see the reward you're working toward.

Once you reach your initial goal keep going. Make another and another and reward yourself for your effort and progress each time. Little by little. One step at a time.

FITNESS COMMITMENT CONTRACT

I, _____, commit to exercising at least 3

days per week by engaging in the following activities:

_____

My Responsibilities:

1. I will eat a balanced, healthy diet that aligns with my fitness goals.

2. I will adhere to my 3-day (or more) per week fitness routine.

My Specific Goals:

_____

Reward for Achieving My Goals (Make it tangible):

Upon reaching my fitness goals, I will reward myself

with:_____

Consequences for Not Meeting Goals: (How will you handle not meeting your goals

without giving up the program?)

_____

Timeline for Completion:

aim to achieve my goals by which date(s): _____

Accountability:

I understand that consistency is key. If I encounter setbacks, I will adjust my plan as

needed and reach out for support from my coach or friends.

Signed: _____ Date: _____

Coach's/Support Person's Signature: _____ Date: _____

(A friend, family member, or support person who will help hold you accountable)

CHAPTER REFLECTION

Date: _____

What did I learn from this chapter?

What will I do differently or apply this week?

How do I feel after completing this chapter?

DRESS FOR SUCCESS

One of the last things people usually think about when starting a fitness program is choosing the right footwear and clothing. Both of these can make working out feel comfortable or torturous. It's already a big enough task to get yourself on a regular routine, you don't need to struggle with overheating, frostbite, or pain in your feet.

Before you take one step exercising, make sure you're wearing appropriate clothing and have the right shoes for your sport and feet. If you're thinking about going shoeless, don't do it! You need shoes to protect your feet and support your body during whatever activity you do. When buying shoes or clothing, here are some things to consider.

CLOTHING

Whether you're going to be exercising in water or climbing a mountain, you need to wear the right clothing. First, remember that your clothing must allow sweat to evaporate or be pulled away from the body. The hotter the weather, the more important this is. When you block the flow of sweat, you force your body to stay warmer than it should. Sweat is your body's way of cooling itself. When that process is interrupted, you could shoot your internal temperature too high and suffer serious damage.

Plastic workout pants and other non-porous materials are dangerous to wear for this reason. In summer, materials like spandex and nylon easily allow evaporation of sweat. In cooler times, cotton is better because it holds heat until you sweat, absorbs the sweat as you perspire, and keeps you warm afterward.

Another function of clothing, especially in colder climates, is insulation. If you're hiking in snow country, dress in layers. That means more than a light T-shirt and heavy jacket. With just a jacket, after you warm up, you only have two options—

leave it on and stay too hot or take it off and get cold. Dressing in layers helps you regulate your insulation. Never let your inner clothing get wet with sweat. Otherwise, if you need to stop, you could get frostbite.

Clothing also needs to protect and support your body throughout your activity. If you're doing water aerobics, don't think you can just jump into a bathing suit and go. Water fitness clothing needs to offer support a swimsuit doesn't provide. A pair of heavy sweats might be perfect for walking on a cold, blustery day, but the same sweats in the heat of summer during an aerobics class could be dangerous.

Wear clothes specifically designed for your sport and season—there's a reason they exist. Seek out an expert in the activity you plan to do and ask what to wear, why, and where to get it. If you can't afford brand names, see what they're made of, what style they are, and choose close imitations or make your own. You'll be more comfortable while moving.

Finally, clothing can get you motivated and excited about exercising! Don't you feel different when you're wearing pajamas compared to when you're all dressed up? Exercise wear works the same way. When you put on your exercise uniform, you play the role. When you "dress up" like an exerciser, you'll be an exerciser.

Activewear can also help you feel good about your achievements. For example, when you've lost a few pounds, getting a new outfit for step class will make you feel great every time you see the results of your hard work in the exercise mirror.

Often, the excitement of getting started overshadows the importance of wearing the right shoes and clothes. Pulling whatever you have out of the drawer and closet may not be the best choice, especially if you're pulling out something you wore 20 years or more ago. Technology has changed. Clothing fabrics have improved. Shoes are lighter and have more cushion than ever before.

Take time to figure out what you'll wear for your activities and get comfortable, affordable shoes. Your feet will be happy, you'll be ready to move, and your new fitness program will be a lot more enjoyable.

SHOES

When your feet hurt, you absolutely won't want to be standing on them. Your first motivation will be to take your shoes off, not finish your workout. Take the time to check with your doctor or chiropractor to see if you have any structural problems that may interfere with the exercise you've chosen. Especially if you've had any kind of foot, knee or back problems before.

For example, if you have knee pain, you'll need a shoe with more stability and motion control to provide good alignment of your foot and ankle to relieve pressure on the knees. If you have one leg much shorter than the other, you may struggle with running or power moves like jumping. In that case you might need a shoe with an adjustable heel lift or custom orthotics to compensate for the difference in leg length. This helps in balancing your posture and reducing strain on your joints. It's worth addressing your specific body mechanics.

Shoes are not cheap, so spend money on the best ones for your feet. Under no circumstances grab the old shoes in your closet that you occasionally use for gardening or yardwork. Old shoes can look brand new but be completely broken down in terms of their support for exercise.

Here's an example. When I first started doing aerobic exercise classes, my feet were a mess. I had no idea what the problem was, only that the morning after exercise, my whole body became stiff and sore—for years. Each morning, I'd wake up wondering why I was still getting sore, even though I was truly in better shape. I didn't feel pain while exercising or afterward, yet I'd wake up barely able to get out of bed. That's not something you expect when you're 24 years old. I saw several chiropractors who analyzed my gait, taped my feet, and did deep stretching. Still, the problem remained. Finally, I saw another chiropractor who recommended soft orthotics for my feet. My feet were pronated and flat. After I got the orthotics, the problem went away overnight. It's amazing how finding the right person to diagnose the problem allowed me to continue with aerobics, which I loved and which eventually became part of my career. It would have been awful to give up my routine and try to find something else I didn't enjoy as much, so I was persistent until I found the answer.

You may need to have that persistence at one point, too. If you don't get the answer from the first medical professional you see, go to another and another if need be. Medical professionals are just people. They don't know everything and each one has their own background, experiences, opinions, and areas of expertise.

Once you know if you have any structural problems, you'll know what type of shoe to look for. Sports podiatrists and online shoe companies can provide a list of shoes and brands best suited for your foot type. For example, flat feet need more motion control or a firmer shoe, while high arches may need a softer, more cushioned shoe. Describe what type of foot you have and what activity you'll be doing. Shoes for walking, aerobics, water activities, tennis, and running all differ. You'll feel better performing your activity if you have the right shoe for it.

When buying shoes, here are some terms to be familiar with:
1. Flexibility – How well the shoe bends at the toes when weight is shifted to the forefoot
2. Comfort – The best feel for your foot type

3. Traction – How smoothly the shoe moves on the exercise surface

4. Stability – How well the shoe anchors the foot firmly in place, no matter the direction of movement

5. Cushion – How well the shoe absorbs shock

6. Fit – The shoe shouldn't be too narrow, wide, large, or small

Here are some buying tips for sport shoes:

1. Don't be pressured into buying any shoe you aren't 100% comfortable and sure about.

2. More expensive doesn't necessarily mean it's the best. You can buy the most expensive shoes in the world, but if they don't fit well and work with your sport, they're a waste of money.

3. No one shoe type is guaranteed to prevent strains or sprains. You have to get the right shoe for you. Proper technique, conditioning, and strengthening exercises are also crucial for preventing injuries.

4. The lighter the shoe, the more easily it will break down, lose support and need replacing.

5. Buy according to the exercise surface (concrete, dirt, wood, carpet, etc.).

6. Wear your shoes only for your activity. You won't have to replace them as often (four months at most). After several months of use, shoes may still look new but no longer have the support and stability you need to exercise safely.

7. Removable insoles are preferable. The shoes are usually better cushioned, and you can add orthotics if needed.

8. Midsoles need to correspond to your body size. Molded EVA (ethyl vinyl acetate) or air cushioning is best for lighter/smaller builds while with TPU (thermoplastic polyurethane) or firmer cushioning systems like PU (polyurethane) offer better durability and support.

9. Buy shoes at the end of the day when your feet are at their largest.

10. Make sure the shoes feel great immediately. If your feet hurt at all, expect it to get worse when you're exercising and your feet swell even more. Athletic shoes should fit like a glove. If they don't feel good after a few days, return them. Retailers will take them back, no problem.

11. If you have feet that are different by a size, go with the larger foot size.

12. Once you've found a shoe that feels great (not just okay) stick with that brand.

13. If you've bought the same shoe more than once and are happy with it try to find the best deal for it online. You'll pay less for it and can afford to replace it more often.

14. Buy according to your fitness level. You won't need top of the line basketball shoes if you're only going to play a few hours a week. If you plan on running everyday though, you'll need a top quality running shoe.

15. If you're going to do several activities, see if there is a shoe that works for more than one. Cross-training varieties in particular can be used for several types of workouts. Check out several kinds before you buy and bring them back if they aren't adaptable to the workouts you were told they would work for.

16. Take care of your shoes too. Let them air out after use and always wear dry, soft, absorbent socks when exercising. If your feet sweat a lot, use foot powder in the shoes. Avoid cleaning them in the washing machine, which will only break them down faster.

LACING

Simple. Just put on your shoes, pull the laces tight and tie. Right? Not so fast. There are multiple ways of lacing shoes each with a different benefit. Choosing the best lacing method depends on your foot shape, activity level, and personal comfort. Proper shoe lacing can make a significant difference in comfort, support, and performance. Included here are several common lacing techniques and their benefits: Experimenting with different techniques can help you find the best one for your feet.

LACING VARIATIONS

Most people don't give much thought to how they lace their shoes, but it can actually make a big difference in your fitness program. The way laces are threaded affects how snugly the shoe holds your foot, how much pressure is placed on the top of your foot, and even how your shoe supports you during movement. Proper lacing can prevent blisters, reduce irritation, and improve comfort, which means you're less likely to cut a workout short or skip it altogether.

Different lacing styles—like the six common ones shown here—can be used to relieve tight spots, create more room, or lock the heel in place, helping you stay consistent and pain-free in your training. If you have a foot issue that these don't address you can search for a lacing option specifically for that. There are various ways to lace shoes if you have toe pain, swollen feet, flat feet and even one specific area that always feels too tight.

1. Standard Lacing

- How: Thread the laces through each pair of eyelets in a crisscross pattern from the bottom to the top.
- Benefits: Provides a balanced fit and is suitable for general activities. It helps distribute pressure evenly across the top of the foot.

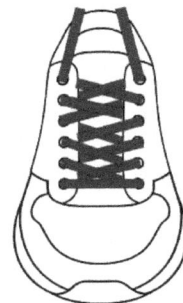

2. Over-Under Lacing

- How: Thread the lace through the eyelets in an over-under pattern to reduce friction and create a smoother feel.
- Benefits: Reduces lace friction, which can be beneficial for longer activities or if you experience discomfort from standard lacing.

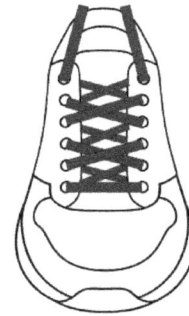

3. Lock Lacing

- How: Create a loop by threading the lace through the top eyelet and then crossing it over to the opposite side. Thread the lace back through the loop.
- Benefits: Helps secure the heel in place, reducing slippage and preventing blisters. Useful for activities involving quick changes in direction or high-impact movements.

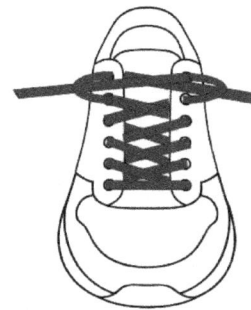

4. Wide Foot Lacing

- How: Skip eyelets to create a wider, more comfortable fit for those with wider feet.
- Benefits: Reduces pressure on the top of the foot and prevents discomfort. Ideal for individuals with broader feet or high arches.

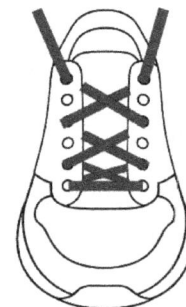

5. High Arch Lacing

- How: Skip the lower eyelets to reduce pressure on the top of your foot, or use additional eyelets higher up for a more secure fit.
- Benefits: Provides a more customized fit for those with high arches, improving comfort and support.

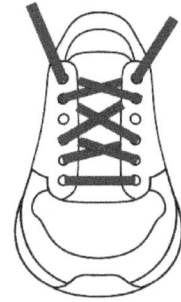

6. Narrow Feet Lacing

- How: Pull the sides of the shoe closer together, ensuring a snug, comfortable fit. This reduces excess room inside the shoe
- Benefits: Improved fit and stability, prevents heel slippage and reduces pain and discomfort

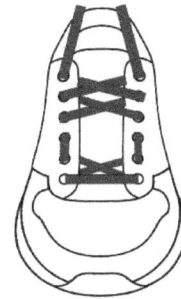

7. Elastic Lacing – Use with any lacing technique

- How: Use elastic laces to allow the shoe to stretch and conform to the foot.
- Benefits: Offers a more flexible fit, making it easier to put on and take off the shoes while providing consistent pressure distribution.

CHAPTER REFLECTION

Date: _____

What did I learn from this chapter?

What will I do differently or apply this week?

How do I feel after completing this chapter?

EQUIPMENT

Aside from the right clothing and shoes, you may be wondering what fitness equipment you might need to get started on your quest for improved fitness. Actually, when you're just starting out you need little to no equipment. Many exercises can be done with just your body weight until you get in better condition and can handle more.

One of the things that I see frequently among newbies, especially in the club/gym, is that they grab weights that they think look "about right". Dumbbells that they think they should be able to maneuver. Unfortunately, people overestimate their abilities. Weights for arm exercises should be very light. For anyone who has not been exercising it's not just the muscle that needs to have the strength to lift the weight, it's also the supporting structures like tendons, ligaments, and stabilizer muscles. That means the potential for getting hurt greatly increases in using any kind of resistance equipment that you aren't accustomed to.

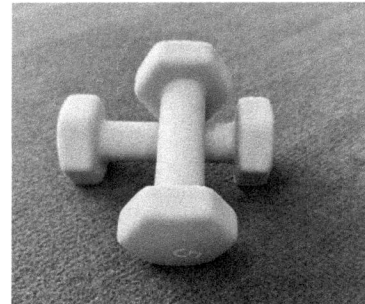

Ankle weights, the same applies. Don't even strap them on until you can easily do all the exercises without them. Give yourself 2-4 weeks without any equipment just to get used to the routine and make sure you are doing all the exercises and stretches properly. At that point you can use soup cans or water bottles for arm work until you have a better idea of what weight is best. For ankle weights, start with the lightest ones or get a pair that is adjustable so that you can remove/insert the weight pouches to achieve the right load. Then you can grow with them over time.

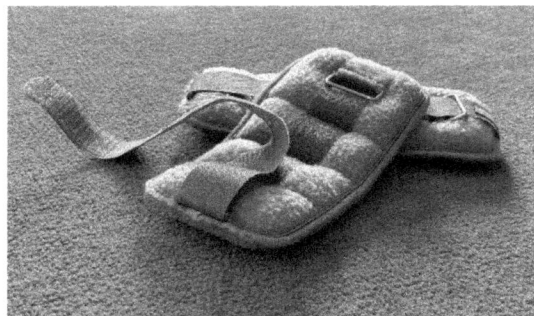

Many people enjoy working out with tubing/bands. Those are resistance items but very light weight. Tubing works by creating tension as you pull on it. It provides a little different type of resistance training in that the amount of tension changes throughout the movement. For example, on a bicep curl the resistance will be harder as the arm raises, where the most load will be felt at the top of the movement. This is in contrast to regular weights where the weight load is the same at the top, bottom or middle of the movement. Regular weights are considered constant resistance. Props that stretch (tubing, bands, and some gym machines) are considered variable resistance.

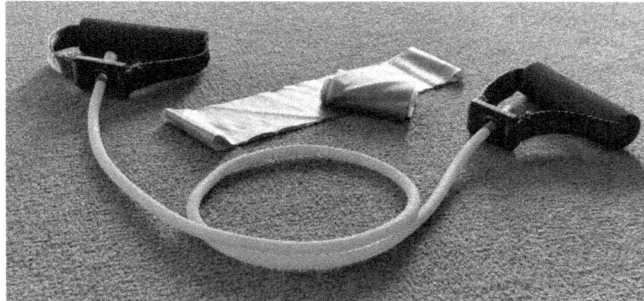

As a general rule, variable resistance is considered safer for beginning exercisers as the load is hardest at the point at which the muscle is strongest. It also works the muscles in both directions (up and down, known as concentric and eccentric movements). These exercises are more like real life movements making it more applicable for improving daily activities and coordination.

There are a number of other beginner friendly props and tools that can assist you in getting more out of your routine. One item I highly recommend is called a stretch out strap. It helps assist during stretching routines, especially if you have tight muscles and are not flexible. The strap has multiple loops on it so that you can place one on a foot and grab hold of the other end with your hands. If you can't touch your toes or have pain while stretching, this is a great tool to help

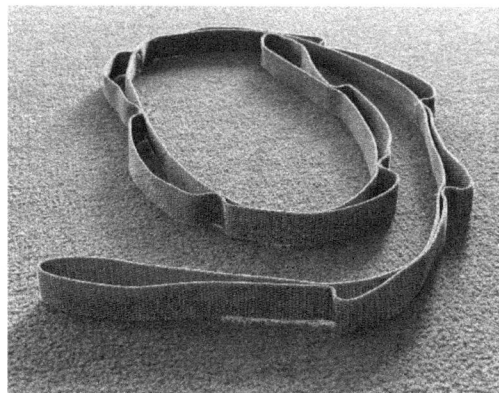

improve flexibility without strain or stress. If you don't have one no worries, you can use a dog leash (stick the clip end through the handle loop to create an end loop) or long towel.

Stability balls (also known as a Swiss ball, exercise ball, or fitness ball) are great for improving balance. If you sit all day they can even become your office chair.

Stability balls are large, inflatable balls made out of elastic material. They're tough enough to support your full body weight and help you develop better balance as the surface is unstable. Stability balls are great for all types of exercise – strength, flexibility, balance and injury rehabilitation.

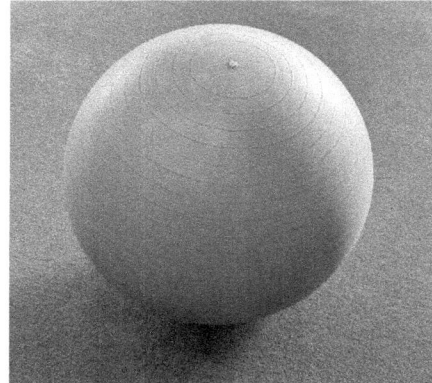

There are many more fitness gadgets out there. Some work really well to make working out fun and effective while others are useless. When you're just getting started stick with basics like what I have mentioned above. Later, once your body is accustomed to exercise and you develop proper exercise technique, you can advance to using other items like steps, foam rollers and sliders. At that point, they'll add variety and keep your workouts exciting. But for now, keep it safe and simple.

CHAPTER REFLECTION

Date: _____

What did I learn from this chapter?

What will I do differently or apply this week?

How do I feel after completing this chapter?

SMART CHOICES IN TRAINERS AND CLASSES

Whether you plan to develop your own fitness program, look for a personal trainer, or join a club, you'll need some guidelines for forming and critiquing the program that would work best for you. What should you look for when choosing a trainer? What about finding the right fitness instructor? Or, what if you're a do-it-yourselfer? How do you set up your own program from step one on? Unless you've been boning up on exercise physiology and anatomy, chances are you're not going to know a whole lot about what to do or why. You're also not going to be sure of what things are important to look for in a trainer or instructor. By using the guidelines that follow you should be able to come up with a sound fitness routine and make qualified choices.

In the United States, personal trainers and fitness instructors are not regulated by a central authority or government body in the same way that some professions (like doctors or nurses) are licensed. That means you have to do your part in finding someone knowledgeable who is the right fit for you.

FINDING A QUALIFIED PERSONAL TRAINER

Working with a certified personal fitness trainer (often referred to as C.P.F.T.) is one of the most expensive ways to get fit but it's also one of the most effective. The trainer is there for you, and only you. They will design the program around your goals and what you can safely do. By focusing on you, technique is perfected and you may try harder just by being the center of attention. Equipment isn't usually something you must have since the trainer has whatever is needed. If you're a private person, you'll like it because you don't have to leave the comfort of your own home or interact with large groups. If you're an outgoing person, there are good trainers at many gyms.

The number one thing you want to think about when searching for a trainer is this: Does the person have the experience dealing with someone of my fitness level? If you're the average person, trying to become fit, you need to find a trainer that works with people like yourself. If you're 70, never exercised a day in your life and are afflicted with arthritis you need someone with experience in those areas. Whatever your physical condition, look for a trainer who is experienced in dealing with issues important to you (motivational, physical, whatever).

Personal trainers will boast all kinds of achievements and credentials. What it all boils down to is do they have what it takes to help you? How much do they know about specific problems or concerns you have?

To find a certified trainer, try visiting the website of the following organizations. They have referral services on their websites that can help you find certified trainers in your area. Here's a list of some of the more credible organizations that refer trainers to individuals:

1. American Council on Exercise (ACE)

ACE has a "Find a Trainer" feature on their website that allows individuals to search for certified trainers based on location and specialties.

2. National Academy of Sports Medicine (NASM)

NASM provides a directory to help individuals find certified trainers. You can search for trainers by location and training specialties.

3. American College of Sports Medicine (ACSM)

ACSM offers a "Find a Trainer" directory on their website that connects individuals with ACSM-certified trainers in their area.

4. National Strength and Conditioning Association (NSCA)

NSCA provides a certification directory where individuals can find NSCA-certified trainers, particularly those with strength and conditioning expertise.

5. International Sports Sciences Association (ISSA)

ISSA offers a "Find a Trainer" tool to help individuals connect with ISSA-certified trainers.

Take care in selecting your trainer based on other points as well - like how comfortable you feel with them, their references, opinions, past experience, etc. Being certified doesn't guarantee a trainer knows what they're doing any more than a medical license can promise the doctor you choose isn't a quack. You can also check academic background too. Ask if they have a degree in physiology or kinesiology for example.

Before hiring anyone, make sure you're comfortable, like the trainer, and like the program they're going to have you do. Is the trainer enthusiastic, sensitive, good at communicating and committed to their own personal health? What about knowledge of various workout equipment? All of these factors directly influence what you'll get out of the training sessions.

CHOOSING A QUALIFIED FITNESS INSTRUCTOR

Fitness instructors can be anyone. And I mean anyone. Someone who works a full time job and dabbles in teaching a class or two mostly for their own fitness level. Stay at home moms who want a few extra dollars. Even an energetic person who formerly took part in the club's classes. I'd much rather take a class from a person studying physical therapy than from a 17 year-old classmate. You are entrusting this person with your physical well-being. You expect them to know an enormous amount about fitness and exude that during class and afterwards.

In other words, almost anyone can step out on the exercise floor and teach. Usually facilities have their own regulations for teaching or set up their own training programs. This doesn't necessarily mean that you'll get a good instructor though. There are many certification organizations for fitness instructors throughout the country. These are the top, credible organizations for aerobics instructors. All of them have been established for decades:

1. **American Council on Exercise (ACE) - Group Fitness Instructor**

   Use the "Find a Trainer" feature on their website that allows individuals to search for ACE-certified group fitness instructors and personal trainers based on location and specialties.

2. **AFAA (Athletics and Fitness Association of America) - Primary Group Exercise Certification**

   AFAA offers a "Find an AFAA Instructor" directory where individuals can search for certified group fitness instructors in their area.

3. **National Academy of Sports Medicine (NASM) - Group Fitness Instructor**

   NASM has a "Find a Trainer" directory that also includes group fitness instructors, allowing individuals to locate certified instructors based on location and specialties.

4. **International Sports Sciences Association (ISSA) - Group Fitness Instructor**

   ISSA offers a "Find a Trainer" tool to help individuals connect with certified group fitness instructors.

5. **National Exercise Trainers Association (NETA) - Group Exercise Instructor Certification**

   NETA provides a directory to find certified group exercise instructors, allowing individuals to search by location.

6. **Fitness & Exercise Association of America (FEAA) - Group Fitness Instructor Certification**

   FEAA offers a directory of certified instructors, making it easy for individuals to find group fitness professionals.

Naturally, you'll find fitness instructors in many more places than clubs. Park and Recreation facilities, small studios, private Zumba Classes, Jazzercise, Dance, Yoga, Barre, Pilates, Kickboxing, Aqua Fitness and more. Any instructor can be good or crummy - it just depends on how much they care and continue to learn.

It's also important to inquire about what other credentials the instructor may have like First Aid, CPR, Basic Lifesaving, etc. I'm sure you'd feel a lot more comfortable exercising with someone you could trust in a medical emergency.

Next, observe classes taught by any and all instructors that you plan on working out with. Watch carefully for contraindicated movements, which are pictured in Appendix 1. If you see any of the movements shown DO NOT sign up or take classes from that individual. You could simply select an alternate movement for those that are dangerous but, I feel strongly that instructors who use any of these exercises in a mixed class are not up to date with current fitness news in general. They may do other more dangerous exercises that are not as easy for you to spot and modify.

Also, each class should have a clear warm-up section. Going back to our car, imagine you're about to drive your car on an icy cold morning. If you hop in and immediately rev the engine to full speed, what happens? The engine struggles, and it may not perform efficiently or could even be damaged. Obviously, it's best to let it idle for a few minutes. This allows the oil to circulate, the engine components to warm up, and the car to get ready for a smooth ride.

Similarly your body needs a warmup before exercising. That means the first 10 minutes should not include strenuous movements. The idea of the warmup is to get the blood circulating and the muscles ready for harder work If you see high knee lifts, fast moves using arms and legs forcefully or lots of squatting forget it - if this is the warm-up what's going to follow? Also, if you see jumping (jump rope too) or running in the warm-up, regardless of the type of class don't join. Those moves are stressful enough when done with fully prepared muscles - the last thing you need is to try to perform them while cold.

Finally, steer away from anyone who uses ballistic stretching. Ballistic stretching involves bouncing while in a stretch and can lead to torn muscle fibers. Safe stretches are held motionless for 30-60 seconds.

Instructors today are getting better and better. Qualified ones can be found in a variety of places - not solely health clubs. If you really don't like the club scene look at parks and recreation departments, local churches, community centers, and in the newspaper for other private groups. Sometimes you'll find better instructors in these places because they generally run their own programs and are personally committed to and interested in their clientele.

Watch both the instructor and the class members. Do they look like they are enjoying the class or is it a grueling experience? Use the Instructor Critique Form at the end of the chapter to help you find a knowledgeable and competent teacher. You don't have to take the form with you, just fill it out after you leave the facility.

If you join a class and find out you don't understand how to do certain exercises or why, ask the instructor. If you don't get adequate information find another teacher. You are putting in your time and money in good faith. Settling for a subpar instructor is not worth endangering your health.

Unfortunately, more times than not, clubs don't offer instructors enough money or incentives to attract those highly qualified. Not being paid enough money to buy clothes, shoes, music, insurance, continuing education, and other equipment makes it hard to attract top notch teachers. It's no wonder why clubs have long had the reputation of featuring young, bouncy, spacey girls as their aerobics instructors. The old saying is true - you get what you pay for. When you pay $10 a month on a club membership you probably aren't going to find expert aerobics instruction.

CHOOSING THE RIGHT CLUB / ROUTINE

Forking out a large sum of money on a club membership doesn't automatically mean you're going to get fit, even if you attend regularly. When utilizing the machines and weights you absolutely need to be sure your workout is specific to your goals. For example, say you want to use the cardio equipment for 30 or more minutes for your aerobic, fat-burning exercise. The club has signs posted that there is a 15 minute time limit on cardio equipment. If that rule is indeed enforced you will not be able to get enough aerobic activity on the machines to help you reach your goals. You also won't get many benefits if you have to wait around so long to use the free weights that you end up leaving before you work all the muscle groups. If you don't know how to use one of the machines, most have a QR code on them that will explain exactly what to do. Look for the QR code if no one is available to help.

A good general routine/class for improving all the above aspects of fitness would include a slow warm-up consisting of light movement followed by cardiovascular or aerobic work within your target heart rate range (min. 20 minutes), strengthening exercises for upper and lower body by weights or other resistance methods (15 minutes), and a cooldown period for deeper stretching and relaxation (10 minutes). To maximize your time, choose a class that addresses all these components otherwise you'll have to supplement the missing ones on your own. Many classes focus on one aspect like aerobics (line dancing, step) or strength (bodysculpting). If you enjoy doing them great - just make sure you incorporate what's missing into your other workouts. Use the Workout Assessment Form provided at the end of the chapter to help you assess the class(es) you're interested in joining. Familiarize yourself with the questions and then answer them after you observe the program.

DEVELOPING YOUR OWN PERSONALIZED PROGRAM

Maybe you're set on designing your own routine. If so, we need to go back to the four components of fitness described in Chapter 2. As mentioned earlier, unless you incorporate cardiovascular endurance, muscular endurance, muscular strength, and flexibility, your workout won't be a balanced one capable of providing you with a totally fit body. Below are Steps To Planning Your Workout.

You'll find out why each of the above components is really necessary and how to make them a part of your workout plan.

STEPS TO PLANNING YOUR WORKOUT

1) WARM-UP

Always remember to take the time to warm up. The first 5-10 minutes of your routine should ALWAYS have a warm-up to prepare your body for what is ahead. You'll feel better during the exercise and afterwards. Start by just moving around. You can slowly walk, march, create different foot movements, whatever - just get your body moving and circulating blood. Save the stretching for the end of your workout.

2) CARDIOVASCULAR ENDURANCE

When talking about improved cardiovascular function, the one type of exercise vital to the process is aerobic exercise. Aerobic exercise is activity which is done in the presence of oxygen. In other words, any activity requiring you to use the largest muscles in the body (legs) at a rate in which you feel yourself starting to breathe heavier and sweat. Energy for aerobic activity is produced slowly but is unlimited in amount. Aerobic exercise would include lower intensity, longer duration type activities such as walking, biking, jogging, swimming, cross country skiing, or aerobic exercise classes. When the aerobic activity is carried out for more than 20 consecutive minutes, fat is burned as the primary fuel source. It may even be burned sooner than that, especially in trained exercisers. By gradually increasing the rate oxygen is pumped to the heart and lungs, the cardiovascular and respiratory systems become stronger. Aerobic exercise has also been shown to be effective for reducing high blood pressure, high blood cholesterol, stress, depression and other health issues.

152

When choosing your aerobic activity choose the form with the least amount of impact. When I say "impact" I'm referring to the forces placed on your feet when doing the activity. For example, a slide board would be considered a non-impact activity just as would swimming and biking. Non-impact just means you're not placing your normal body weight on your feet. The feet either don't come off the floor or never come in contact with it.

Low-impact activity places about 1-2 times of your body weight on the feet each time you step. Low-impact exercises would be walking, trampoline, stepping, water aerobics, and skating. Add jumping or running motions and you have what is called high-impact.

High-impact puts 3-4 times your body weight on the feet each time you land on them. Examples would be running, hopping, jumping rope, soccer, and tennis. High-impact exercise is generally associated with more injury and is not recommended when beginning a program. If you love tennis and jogging don't fret. As long as you don't have any physical reason why not to (like being obese or having a back/knee injury), add them a few months into the program after you've strengthened your muscles, ligaments and tendons to absorb the added stress.

By contrast, anaerobic exercise means without the presence of oxygen. This would involve short sudden bursts of energy like that found in weightlifting, calisthenics, sprinting, tennis doubles, football, and baseball. Anaerobic exercise produces energy at a rapid rate but for a brief period of time. This is done at a very high intensity, for a short time (from a few seconds to a few minutes). Although anaerobic exercise is good for building strength and quick bursts of energy, it doesn't condition the cardiovascular system as well as aerobic exercise.

If your goals involve losing fat or bolstering your cardiovascular system, the preferred method is aerobic exercise. So, how can you tell if the activity you want to do is aerobic or not? Easy. If it requires stop-and-go movement it's anaerobic.

Continuous, steady activity using the legs is surely aerobic. Some activities can be either. For example, dancing can be aerobic if done moderately without stopping for 20 or so minutes or it can be anaerobic if done wildly for several minutes followed by rest. Yard work can be aerobic if you continually mow the yard at a quick pace for 20 or more minutes. It can be anaerobic if you spend the time lifting heavy bricks, pottery or digging. A circuit training class can be aerobic if done without breaks with every other station using large leg muscles for movement. Or it can be anaerobic if each station works one muscle at a time with short rests in between.

3) MUSCULAR STRENGTH / ENDURANCE

Muscular strength just means how much weight a particular muscle can resist. When you're carrying groceries how many bags can you hold at a time? Strength is important for more than just carrying groceries. As we age, we gradually lose strength. According to Doctor Wayne Westcott, adults who do no strength training at all lose an average of five pounds of muscle every ten years of life. Combine that with the fact that after high school the average non-exercising person will gain at least one pound a year for each year of life and you'll see how easy it is to end up with a pot belly well before middle age. Keeping active and fit can also protect against many injuries associated with aging.

Perhaps the greatest argument for strength training is what it does for your metabolism. As you develop more and more muscle you become firmer and tighter (not necessarily BIGGER). That denser muscle tissue needs to burn a lot of calories to keep itself nourished. The end result? Your metabolism goes up. Yep, it goes up and stays up - even when you're not working out. By having more muscle you can enjoy the benefit of having extra calories burned all day long. And, when calories burned are greater than calories taken in, you lose weight. That's a plus when you're trying to get rid of fat.

To make sure your program offers a strength training segment you'll need to incorporate some type of resistance equipment like free weights, tubing, bands, or machines. This can be as inexpensive as a simple flat elastic band or as costly as the top of the line weight machine. Totally up to you. The results will be the same.

Locate the sample weight training routines located in Appendix 2 to help you get started. There are two different programs to choose from. All are pictured with free weights since it's a lot easier to buy a couple of pairs of dumbbells than a whole weight room set up. If you already have other equipment, many of the movements will be the same.

Start with one program and stick with it for six to eight weeks. Then, go on to another for the next six to eight weeks. Alternate back and forth. The variety will constantly challenge your muscles and offer you the best results. If an exercise feels uncomfortable, use the corresponding exercise from the second plan instead.

Muscular endurance is increased through strength training. For example, if you can do 1 dumbbell fly (strength) with 20 lbs. in each hand you should be able to do 10 flyes (endurance) with 75% of 20 lbs. When you improve to lift 30 lbs. once, you should be able to perform 10 flyes with 75% again or 22 lbs. When you increase muscular strength, muscle endurance is increased too.

What's the point? Well, besides a higher metabolism you need strength training for several other important reasons. One, more muscle also means a more sculpted looking body. It's the muscle tissue which adds shape and definition to the way you look and most people prefer a sculpted look to simply being thin. Two, in terms of injury, a strong body with all muscles equally balanced leads to fewer injuries and faster injury recovery. Lastly, endurance allows you to perform a given movement over and over again (like walking, shoveling, climbing a ladder, etc.). You can probably think of many day to day activities that would be easier for you if you had a bit more endurance. Your workout should include anywhere from 10-20 minutes of strength and endurance work.

4) FLEXIBILITY

This simply refers to the range of motion around a joint. Without adequate flexibility you become more prone to injuries, especially as you get older. Stretching keeps each joint's range of motion at its fullest potential. For example, say you have a neck problem and the tight muscles in the area inhibit you from being able to use your left arm to reach as fully as the right arm. With proper stretching, the difference between the two arms should slowly diminish. So will the probability that you'll get injured by suddenly trying to reach beyond your limit. Any program you embark upon should have a stretching section devoted to improving flexibility. Stretching is best done after you've exercised when muscles are warm and more pliable.

The kind of stretching you did when you were young like bouncing to the ground and touching your toes is out! That is a ballistic stretch and is neither the safe nor preferable method of increasing flexibility. The body has a protective mechanism which will actually pull the muscle back rapidly if it senses that it is being stretched too far. When you perform a ballistic stretch, that mechanism (golgi tendon organ) contracts the stretched muscle to protect it from what it senses to be dangerous. It works much like when you nod off while sitting. Your head starts to tilt to the side. As the neck muscles get to the point of overstretching, the golgi tendon organ quickly pulls them back up. You become startled, wake up and your head is erect.

A safer, more effective way to stretch is to use static stretches or those which are held. Put both your arms out in front of you. Overlap one hand with the other and press both arms straight out in front of you. Round your shoulders forward and hold. That is a static stretch. If you hold the stretch long enough (60 seconds) you'll notice the muscles in the upper back get to a point at which they actually let go and stretch further. Static stretching does not pose a risk of tearing or injuring muscles and will lead to greater gains in flexibility.

There's also what is called active and passive stretching. Active stretching refers to stretches which are done while moving. Instead of jerking, ballistic type movements, active stretching is that done slowly vs. forcefully. For example, reaching your arms overhead and bringing them back down slowly several times. Going through actual motions you will be using during your workout but at a slower, gentler pace will warm you up and stretch muscles. Passive stretching involves holding one particular stretch without movement. If you're sitting in a chair put your right ankle on your left knee. Lean forward. Hold yourself in that position at which you feel tightness. That's a passive static stretch.

If you're designing your own routine, start with the stretch plans suggested in Appendix 3. One plan is done standing, the other one sitting or on the floor. They should be comfortable for most new students to perform. Choose one to start with and rotate them. Eventually you'll know every stretch that can target the muscle you want and you won't need the plans anymore. Just make sure you cover all the muscle groups listed. As you progress you can challenge yourself with other stretches not included here, but for now stick with these. They safely address the major muscle groups you need to stretch. If any one stretch feels too uncomfortable to do, substitute it with the stretch for the same muscle from the other stretch plan.

I must emphasize one thing about stretching (this actually applies to the rest of your program too). Everybody is different and what may be comfortable for you may be painful to someone else. Listen to your body and don't do any stretches that produce pain. Age, injury, and inactivity can limit the types and positions of stretches you'll feel comfortable in. Proper stretching should feel uncomfortable if you lengthen the muscle to its limit. It should never, never, never, feel agonizing. I've witnessed many yoga classes that involve movements that are downright dangerous, especially to beginning students. If you're interested in yoga, learn everything you can about it first and analyze the moves. Don't do any stretches which require you to stand and lean forward without the weight of your upper body supported. The lower back can be damaged permanently by doing unsupported forward flexion of this kind. Never force a stretch and never quickly switch from one stretch to another. Always use the last 10 minutes of your workout for stretching.

After you've finished designing your workout program, fill out the Workout Assessment Form at the end of the chapter. This will help you locate any problem areas in the design of your routine.

ONLINE APPS AND PROGRAMS

Your best bet for choosing a good quality fitness app is to look at the background of the person who created it. There are thousands of exercise apps and online workouts to choose from and to the unsuspecting consumer they all look good. Beware though - many of them contain questionable exercises for those just starting out or are strictly a scheme to make fast money.

Numerous celebrities put out fitness videos because you are familiar with them and most likely want to have their looks or shape. Stay away from the celebrity choices. Instead look for people who've been in the fitness industry for many years. These people have devoted their lives to helping people get and stay fit. They've done their homework and know what is safe and what is dangerous. They also are more likely to have content geared specifically for beginners. A beginner workout is one that isn't going to be too strenuous, contain too many complicated moves and is easy to understand and follow.

If you're the kind of person who can stay motivated using digital content select several workouts and alternate them. Not only will you stay more interested but also challenge your muscles in a different way daily. Doing the same routine day after day soon becomes easy for your muscles to adapt to. Variety is very important to think about along with making sure you have uninterrupted exercise time.

If you're still not sure about which would be appropriate for you stay away from titles with the words "Power", "Challenge", "Blast", and "Creative". Avoid any workout that is high-impact or involves running motions. You also probably won't want the advanced choreography of funk, hip hop or street dance style either. Unless you're an aspiring choreographer, you'll get too frustrated. Don't be afraid to try multiple apps and workouts. When you find one you really feel good with, buy it or similar ones created by the same person.

INSTRUCTOR CRITIQUE FORM

1. Does the instructor show a caring for students?

2. Does the instructor interact with students and know their names?

3. Does the instructor look around the room and teach for members as opposed to staring into the mirror and teaching for their own benefit?

4. Does the instructor perform a gentle warm-up moving all the major body parts?

5. Does the instructor follow the class format (Ex., is low-impact without running and jumping moves)?

6. Does the atmosphere feel warm and lively instead of cold and sterile?

7. Does the instructor build the aerobic section gently as opposed to simply going all out?

8. Do they offer alternative movements for those not able to work as hard or who don't have adequate coordination?

9. Is the instructor encouraging as opposed to intimidating?

160

10. Does the instructor offer personal help to those having a difficult time or who are incorrectly doing the motions?

11. Is the instructor focused on the exercise experience instead of the choreography?

12. Do they have students take their heart rate?

13. Do they gradually take a few minutes to transition from hard aerobic activity to slow floor exercise?

14. Does the instructor move around and help students during floor work?

15. Does the instructor end class with a relaxing section with slow moves and stretches?

16. Did they educate about different muscles or fitness concepts?

17. Does their class look like fun?

While observing an instructor you should be able to answer all the above. The more "yes" answers, the greater the chance you've located an excellent teacher. If you answered "no" to more than a few, look around more. Even if you have to pay a class fee for observing, it's well worth the full cost of a membership that you don't use.

WORKOUT ASSESSMENT FORM

(For classes or individual routines)

1. Is there a warm-up?

2. Is it approximately 10 minutes long?

3. Does it start out slow and gradually increase in intensity?

4. Is the warm-up done without any jumping or running?

5. Is there an aerobic section?

6. Is it at least 20 minutes of continuous activity?

7. Is the aerobic section at a pace you can handle for the entire time?

8. Does the aerobic section end with a heart rate check?

9. Does the aerobic section end with a gradual cooling down as opposed to a complete stop of all movement?

10. Are there strength exercises using weights, bands, or other resistance products?

11. Are all the major muscles clearly worked (i.e.., major arm muscles, major leg muscles, abdominals)?

12. Is the strength section at least 10-15 minutes long?

13. Are there stretching exercises at the end for flexibility?

14. Are all stretches held at their tightest point as opposed to being bounced?

If you answered "No" to any of the above, go back and refine your program until you find a "Yes" answer to each. If you're assessing a class which is missing specific criteria, list below how you plan on fixing the weak areas. For example, the class is completely aerobic, no strength work whatsoever. You can solve the problem by adding 10 minutes of strength work on your own before the class cools down and ends, then stretch on your own immediately following.

CHAPTER REFLECTION

Date: _____

What did I learn from this chapter?

What will I do differently or apply this week?

How do I feel after completing this chapter?

INJURIES

It would be great if each one of us could start the same fitness program and do each and every exercise without some kind of pain, discomfort or danger. Unfortunately, that's not the case. I must stress the importance of "listening to your body" here. If/when you perform any activity that causes you any pain, stop! I'm not talking about the kind of sensation that lets you know you're working your muscles. "Pain" can be an uncomfortableness from doing the exercise right or a dangerous type from stressing part of your body to the point of injury. I'm referring to a distinctive type of discomfort that should send a red light flashing in your head that something is not right.

Sometimes though, no matter how careful you are or how slow you go, you may sustain an injury. Injuries often happen when first starting out. Keep in mind that pretty much everyone who exercises will be injured at one time or another. It doesn't mean it's time to throw in the towel. After all, an occasional pulled muscle is worth all those long term benefits. It does mean that you need to take time for the injury to heal so that you can get back to your routine as soon as possible. If not, you'll continue to see repeated episodes of the injury and over time it will cause you to miss many more days.

It's also vital to determine what caused the injury. Was it from overdoing it? Having the wrong shoes? Not knowing how to safely use the equipment? Having a personal trainer push you beyond your limits? Finding out the cause of the injury will help prevent you from experiencing it again.

In the case of most injuries the best initial plan of action is REST (Rest, Ice, Compression, Elevation). Treat the injury with ice, not heat, wrap it with a compression bandage and elevate it above heart level. Below are some of the most common injuries related to fitness. Look them over so that if you ever suspect you have one, you'll be able to identify it.

1. Muscle Strains

- **What it is**: Overstretching or tearing of muscle fibers, usually caused by pushing too hard too soon or not warming up properly.

- **Common areas**: Lower back, hamstrings, calves, shoulders.

2. Joint Sprains

- **What it is**: Stretching or tearing of ligaments around joints, usually from improper form or overuse.

- **Common areas**: Ankles, knees, wrists.

3. Knee Pain (Patellofemoral Pain Syndrome)

- **What it is**: Pain around the kneecap, often due to weak muscles, improper footwear, or overuse during running or squats.

- **Causes**: Poor form, jumping into high-impact activities without preparation.

4. Shin Splints

- **What it is**: Pain along the shinbone (tibia), often due to running on hard surfaces or increasing workout intensity too quickly.

- **Causes**: Inadequate footwear, poor running technique, or overtraining.

5. Plantar Fasciitis

- **What it is**: Inflammation of the thick tissue on the bottom of the foot, usually from improper footwear or increasing physical activity suddenly.

- **Causes**: Poor foot support, rapid increase in activity, high-impact exercises like running. Footwear devices to help treat plantar fasciitis are widely available online.

6. Lower Back Pain

- **What it is**: Strain or stress on the muscles, ligaments, or discs in the lower back, often from improper lifting techniques or weak core muscles.
- **Causes**: Bad form during weightlifting, excessive bending, or poor posture during exercises.

7. Tendinitis

- **What it is**: Inflammation of the tendons, often due to overuse or repetitive movements.
- **Common areas**: Shoulders, elbows (tennis elbow), knees, and Achilles tendon.

8. Pulled Groin

- **What it is**: Strain in the muscles of the inner thigh, often from sudden movements like lunges, stretches, or side-to-side activities.
- **Causes**: Lack of flexibility or improper warm-up before engaging in dynamic activities.

9. Shoulder Injuries (Rotator Cuff Strain)

- **What it is**: Damage or irritation to the muscles and tendons in the shoulder joint, typically from improper lifting techniques or overuse.
- **Causes**: Overhead exercises, poor form, or lifting too much weight.

10. Wrist Injuries

- **What it is**: Strain on the wrist joints or tendons, often from poor hand positioning during push-ups, planks, or lifting weights.

- **Causes**: Incorrect form or sudden increase in activity.

Injuries aren't always your fault. Knowing what can cause some of them can help you avoid those things that contribute to them.

CHAPTER REFLECTION

Date: _____

What did I learn from this chapter?

What will I do differently or apply this week?

How do I feel after completing this chapter?

REST AND RELAXATION

Getting enough rest (meaning sleep) and making time for relaxation are often confused, but they serve very different roles in your overall health. Both are essential for achieving your fitness goals and losing weight, but they affect your body and mind in distinct ways.

REST

Rest refers to sleep, which is your body's natural recovery process. It's during sleep that your muscles repair, your immune system strengthens, and your brain processes and stores information from the day. For adults, the optimal amount of sleep is typically 7 to 9 hours per night. Less than that and your body doesn't get enough time, which can lead to fatigue, reduced performance, and a higher risk of injury.

When it comes to weight loss, sleep is critical. Poor sleep disrupts your hormones, particularly ghrelin (which increases hunger) and leptin (which tells you when you're full). If you're sleep-deprived, you're more likely to feel hungry throughout the day and crave high-calorie, unhealthy foods. Plus, you're less likely to have the energy or motivation to work out. Simply put, not getting enough sleep makes it much harder to stick to your fitness and weight-loss goals.

Consuming caffeine before bed may impair your ability to get to sleep as will using your bed for activities other than sleep, like scrolling on your phone or working on a laptop.

RELAXATION

While sleep is about physical recovery, relaxation is more about mental recovery. Relaxation helps manage stress, which, if left unchecked, can derail your efforts to lose weight. Stress triggers the release of cortisol, a hormone that, when elevated over long periods, encourages fat storage—particularly in the abdominal area.

Relaxation techniques help to lower cortisol levels and reduce the overall stress load on your body. Some effective relaxation practices include:

- **Meditation:** Even just a few minutes of quiet focus on your breathing or heartbeat can calm your mind and reduce stress.
- **Deep Breathing:** Taking slow, deep breaths for a few minutes can immediately lower your stress levels.
- **Guided Visualization:** Listen to a guided meditation that leads you through calming imagery, such as a peaceful beach or serene forest.
- **Progressive Relaxation:** Tense and then relax each muscle group in your body, starting from your toes and working your way up. Focus on the difference between tension and relaxation.
- **Reading:** A good book can take your mind off your worries and give you a mental break.
- **Journaling:** Writing down your thoughts can help you process your emotions and release stress.
- **Nature Walks:** Being outdoors, especially in green spaces or at the beach, has been shown to lower stress and improve mental well-being. Sunlight exposure increases vitamin D, very important for mental health.

Regular relaxation helps you stay mindful and balanced. It gives you the mental clarity to make better decisions—whether it's choosing a healthy snack or finding the motivation to go for a workout. Without relaxation, stress can build up, making it harder to stick to healthy habits and ultimately hindering weight loss.

Both rest and relaxation are important. If you prioritize sleep but ignore relaxation, you're missing out on mental benefits that can help you handle stress. Conversely, if you focus only on relaxation but don't get enough sleep, your body won't fully recover physically. You need both to achieve a well-rounded approach to fitness and weight loss. Sleep restores your body, while relaxation recharges your mind.

By ensuring you get seven to nine hours of sleep each night and incorporating relaxation techniques into your day, you'll reduce stress, make better food choices, and stay motivated to work out. Together, these habits keep your body and mind in peak condition, setting you up for success on your fitness and weight loss journey.

So, integrate both rest and relaxation as key parts of your routine. They're the foundation of a healthier, more balanced lifestyle that will support your long-term fitness goals. The following page includes a Sample Relaxation Script that you can record in your own soft, slow voice. Listen to it when you have a few minutes and need to relax. You can also find a variety of similar pieces with free ambient music available on YouTube. Try searching "Guided Relaxation," "Mindfulness Meditation" and "Deep Relaxation Techniques."

Sample Relaxation Script
(Record using a soft, slow paced voice for playback with ambient music)

Gently guide your mind and body into a state of calm. Find a comfortable position—whether lying down or sitting—and allow your body to settle.

Start by closing your eyes……..take a slow, deep breath in through your nose, feeling your lungs expand………. hold it for a moment……… now, exhale gently through your mouth…………. notice the sensation of the air leaving your body.

Do that again: Inhale slowly, filling your lungs fully………. Hold for just a second…………. and now exhale slowly………. With each exhale, let go of any stress or tension………. Let your body sink a little deeper into comfort.

Now, bring your attention to your body………. notice how it feels in this moment…………. without trying to change anything, just observe…………. is there tightness anywhere?………. a sense of relaxation in some areas?………. just notice how your entire body feels right now.

Take some time to work through each part of your body, releasing tension as you go………. if you feel any discomfort, remember to be gentle with yourself.

Start with your head and face………. as you breathe in, scrunch your facial muscles—squeeze your eyes shut, wrinkle your nose, tighten your jaw............. hold that for a few seconds............. Now, as you exhale, release the tension in your face............ Letting your expression soften completely............ feel any tightness melt away.........your face and all the muscles are totally relaxed.

Now, bring attention to your shoulders and neck.......... inhale deeply and gently shrug your shoulders up toward your ears............. feel the tension in your neck and shoulders.......... hold for a moment............. now, exhale slowly, and let your shoulders drop........... releasing all tension as they relax.......... feel your neck and shoulders soften and expand.

Move your awareness to your arms and hands.......... inhale slowly, and as you do, clench your fists and tighten the muscles in your arms............. hold that for a few seconds............. now, exhale gently as you release the tension in your hands and arms............. let your arms rest softly at your sides............. feel the weight of your arms sinking into relaxation.

Bring your focus to your chest and back now............. take a deep breath in, and gently tighten your chest and upper back muscles.......... hold for a moment............. then exhale slowly, letting go of all tightness in your chest and back..........feel your chest relax, expanding as you breathe easily.

Next, focus on your stomach and lower back........... inhale deeply, gently tightening your stomach muscles.......... hold the tension for a moment........... and as you exhale, let the muscles soften and release...........

Imagine your stomach melting into the surface beneath you............ let your lower back relax completely.

Now bring your attention to your thighs and calves............ take a deep breath in, and gently tighten the muscles in your thighs and calves.......... hold that tension for a few seconds............. and now, as you exhale, let the tension go completely............ feel your legs growing heavy and relaxed.......... sinking deeper into comfort.

Finally, focus on your feet.......... on your next breath in, gently scrunch your toes and tense the muscles in your feet........... hold it for a moment............. and as you exhale, release all the tension in your feet............. let the muscles in your feet go completely limp, allowing them to soften and rest.

Now, take a moment to notice your entire body, from head to toe............ how does it feel compared to when you started?............ with each breath, imagine any remaining tension leaving your body.

Take three more deep breaths, and with each exhale........... feel your body growing more and more relaxed........... like a gentle wave of calmness washing over you.

When you're ready........... slowly bring your awareness back to the present moment.......... gently move your fingers and toes............. feel your body against the surface beneath you.......slowly open your eyes, taking your time to adjust.

You are now relaxed and refreshed.......... ready to carry this sense of calm with you for the rest of the day........... Remember, you can return to this relaxed state anytime you need by focusing on your breath and body.

CHAPTER REFLECTION

Date: _____

What did I learn from this chapter?

What will I do differently or apply this week?

How do I feel after completing this chapter?

WEIGHT LOSS AIDS

DRUGS

Weight loss drugs have been around for decades, but they've always come with risks. In the 1990s, it was Fen-Phen and Ephedra. By the early 2000s, it was Orlistat. In the 2010s, Lorcaserin hit the market. Each of these drugs promised weight loss but carried some heavy baggage: heart valve damage, lung failure, heart attacks, stroke, and cancer were all on the table.

Today's weight loss medications are more advanced, but they're not without their own risks. Some of the most recent popular drugs —Ozempic, Wegovy, Rybelsus, Mounjaro, Qsymia, and Victoza—promise big results by curbing hunger and regulating blood sugar. But, just like those before them, they come with their own set of risks: nausea, vomiting, pancreatitis, increased heart rate, and in some cases, potential thyroid issues and birth defects. These may be the current big names, but weight loss drugs tend to come in waves—new ones appear, old ones fade out, and each generation brings its own claims and concerns. The cycle continues, with new names, new promises, and new risks always on the horizon.

Weight loss drugs aren't for everyone. First, they're used to suppress appetite. That means if you're someone who uses food as a way to cope with or manage emotions rather than eating due to physical hunger, they're likely to have little effect on you. There aren't any drugs that can stop mindless eating, urges to eat comfort foods, or eating to numb feelings.

In addition, they're usually prescribed for people with a BMI of 30 or higher (27 if they've got conditions like diabetes or high blood pressure), so the ideal candidates are those who are severely obese with serious health issues. Even then, these drugs work best when combined with a healthy diet, regular exercise, and behavior changes. They're not a magic fix, and most are approved for short-term use only. We still don't fully understand the long-term effects, so if you decide to take them, consider yourself part of an experiment. The lasting impact won't be known until these drugs are studied for years to come.

The big problem with relying on weight loss drugs is what happens after you stop taking them. Without real lifestyle changes of regular exercise and a balanced diet, the weight usually comes back. And even if you do lose weight, it's only going to last while you're on the drug.

You're also missing out on all the benefits that exercise brings. There's no muscle tone, strength, endurance, flexibility, or mental health boost. You might lose pounds, but you won't gain all those true benefits of living a healthy, active life.

SUPPLEMENTS

Supplements should be used with caution, and it's best to focus on getting them from whole foods rather than relying on pills or powders alone. Here are some vitamins and minerals that can support overall health, metabolism, and energy levels, which might assist with weight management.

1. Vitamin D

How it helps: Low levels of vitamin D are associated with obesity and weight gain. It is believed that vitamin D helps regulate fat cells and the production of hormones like leptin, which signals the brain about hunger and fat storage.

Plant-Based Sources: Sun exposure, fortified plant-based milks/cereals, mushrooms, and supplements.

2. B Vitamins (B12, B6, B1, B2, Niacin, Folate)

How they help: B vitamins play a crucial role in energy metabolism. They help convert food into energy, which is necessary for staying active and maintaining a healthy metabolism. Deficiencies in B vitamins can lead to fatigue, making it harder to stick with an exercise routine.

B12: Often promoted for boosting energy levels. Vegans in particular must take a B12 supplement as their diet without animal products will be missing this important vitamin. A deficiency could lead to permanent nerve damage and serious cognitive problems.

B6: Involved in protein and fat metabolism.

Plant-Based Sources: Whole grains, legumes, leafy greens, nutritional yeast, fortified plant-based foods, and supplements.

3. Vitamin C

How it helps: Vitamin C is an antioxidant that supports the immune system and helps the body burn fat during exercise. Studies suggest that people with adequate vitamin C levels burn more fat during moderate exercise than those with low levels.

Plant-Based Sources: Citrus fruits, berries, bell peppers, broccoli, and supplements.

4. Iron

How it helps: Iron supports the transportation of oxygen in the blood and helps convert nutrients into energy. People who are iron deficient often feel fatigued, which can make it difficult to exercise, potentially contributing to weight gain.

Plant-Based Sources: Lentils, beans, tofu, spinach, pumpkin seeds, quinoa, and fortified foods.

5. Magnesium

How it helps: Magnesium is involved in over 300 biochemical reactions in the body, including energy production, muscle function, and the regulation of blood sugar and insulin levels. It may help reduce belly fat and improve metabolism by regulating glucose and insulin.

Plant-Based Sources: Nuts, seeds, leafy greens, whole grains, and supplements.

6. Calcium

How it helps: Some studies suggest that calcium may help the body break down fat and reduce the storage of fat. It may also regulate how fat cells function and their storage of fats.

Plant-Based Sources: Fortified plant-based milks, tofu made with calcium sulfate, leafy greens (like kale, bok choy), almonds, and supplements.

7. Chromium

How it helps: Chromium is believed to help regulate blood sugar by improving insulin sensitivity. This can reduce sugar cravings and overeating, leading to better weight control.

Plant-Based Sources: Whole grains, broccoli, potatoes, and supplements.

8. Coenzyme Q10 (CoQ10)

How it helps: CoQ10 is involved in energy production within cells. It may support physical performance, especially in people with deficiencies, allowing for more effective exercise, which is key to weight loss.

Plant-Based Sources: Spinach, broccoli, cauliflower, whole grains, legumes, nuts, seeds, and supplements.

9. Omega-3 Fatty Acids

How they help: Omega-3s, particularly EPA and DHA, can reduce inflammation, improve heart health, and regulate fat metabolism. They may also enhance the effects of exercise on weight loss by improving the body's fat-burning ability.

Plant-Based Sources: Flaxseeds, chia seeds, hemp seeds, walnuts, seaweed, algae-based supplements.

10. Zinc

How it helps: Zinc plays a role in appetite regulation and hormone production. Deficiencies in zinc can impair thyroid function, which in turn can slow metabolism and lead to weight gain.

Plant-Based Sources: Beans, lentils, chickpeas, pumpkin seeds, cashews, whole grains, and supplements.

11. Probiotics

How they help: Probiotics are beneficial bacteria that support gut health. Some research suggests that improving gut microbiota can aid in weight management, reduce inflammation, and improve metabolism.

Plant-Based Sources: Plant-based yogurts with live cultures, sauerkraut, kimchi, miso, tempeh, kombucha, and probiotic supplements.

SHAKES AND SNACKS

There are all kinds of substances that people believe will help them lose weight but are simply ineffective. Avoid spending your money on these items as they aren't proven to help in weight loss. The list includes things like cider vinegar, detox teas, green coffee bean extract, capsaicin (in spicy foods), coconut oil, bitter orange, and L-Carnitine.

What about a protein shake instead of a meal? Protein is good to keep you full, right? Skipping meals can slow metabolism, increase hunger, and make it harder to sustain a healthy diet long-term. Regular, balanced meals with protein can be more effective for fat loss. Protein powders can contain a lot of additives and extra calories which is definitely something to steer clear of.

Maybe you just want to have a protein bar now and then. Isn't protein important for muscle growth? As far as protein bars, maybe during or after an endurance event like a 5K but for day-to-day consumption they aren't necessary. You can get the same protein content from eating a healthy peanut butter sandwich. Whatever you can make at home will cost a fraction of what these things cost to purchase. Remember, protein isn't going to turn into muscle. You'll need strength training to build muscle mass and boost your metabolism

If you're thinking about taking any of the above substances think long-term. Are you willing to be on a drug for your lifetime, rely on daily supplements that you could get through a healthy diet or pay for powders/bars that don't give you any better edge than eating right and exercising? Save yourself the expense unless your life depends upon rapid weight loss, in which case the risk may be worth the benefit.

CHAPTER REFLECTION

Date: _____

What did I learn from this chapter?

What will I do differently or apply this week?

How do I feel after completing this chapter?

TESTIMONIALS

It's always inspiring to hear the true feelings of real people. Over the years, I've asked my students to jot down a few sentences about why they exercise and what it does for them. I've enjoyed reading their stories and thank them for sharing their honest thoughts about fitness. Here's what they had to say—I hope their words encourage you in ways I can't.

"To me, the most important benefit of exercise is its stabilizing influence. I find this absolutely essential at this time of my life. In middle age, you go through all kinds of changes - mental, emotional, social, marital, and, of course, physical. Even though many of these changes are exciting and welcome, others are stressful and can be depressing. Exercise gives you a sense of having some control over all this. After class, you feel more calm and able to cope emotionally, more alert mentally, and less tired physically, because you've worked away the stress. And I feel like regular workouts help your body cope better with the hormonal changes - to even out the fluctuations - you go through at this age. In general, exercise gives you reassurance that you're going to be able to keep vital and active, despite growing older."

Jill F.

"Five years ago, my sister invited me to go with her to an aerobics class. Aerobics was the last thing I had in mind when it came to exercise. I was not an athletic person and I felt awful physically whenever I ran, so how was I ever going to be able to do aerobics? The last 5 years have been a wonderful, growing experience for me physically and emotionally. Exercise has helped strengthen my muscles and toned them, I am soon to be 45 years old and have great blood pressure and low cholesterol. But the greatest benefit for me is that

emotionally I have never felt better. I rarely have a down day and find that I enjoy life more. Exercise just makes me feel good!"

Noelle C.

"I signed up for exercise class out of desperation and disgust with my body. In other words, for totally negative reasons. I ran the gamut, spending time, money and effort on everything from health clubs (where larger-size people suddenly become invisible to home equipment, workout tapes, books, psycho and hypno therapy. Still, somehow it just wouldn't all come together. It seemed the harder I tried to control my body, the more out of control my body became. I was miserably at war with myself. So, I signed up immediately when I found an exercise class specially tailored to my needs.

Now, almost a year later, I'm at the other end of the spectrum. I continue to exercise regularly to keep my mind and spirit in synch with my body, to keep myself positively balanced. In other words, for totally positive reasons. It's my time to commune with myself. Losing fat has very little to do with the equation anymore; it's a natural byproduct of getting STRONG, a process that seems invisible at first. It took months to build up the necessary strength inside my body before I could actually see - and feel - that I was STRONG. And, when that happened, my mind no longer tried to rule my body. The obsession was gone.

So, now that my mind and body are equal partners, it's only fair that they get equal time. I continue to love to read. But now I love to exercise too."

Cheryl F.

"Exercise has been a part of a healing restoration process that has taken place within the last year of my life. One year ago I left an abusive marriage, and had to literally re-build my life, my friends, my patterns and interests. Exercise,

188

specifically an aerobics class, provided structure, regular exercise, a sense of community with other women, an outlet for tensions and a sense of well-being to combat feelings of depression. It has definitely been a vital part of a healing process, and one that I treasure a great deal."

Susan A.

"My name is Stephanie. I am a 53 year old woman who weighs 250 pounds. Until January 17, 1994 (Northridge Earthquake Day) I had never exercised a day in my life. After speaking with Michele the week before, I had decided to begin Largercise classes with her no matter what. I have dieted for 30 years and weigh 100 pounds more than when I began so I decided diets are not the way for me to go. I have been exercising 3 times a week since then and can't express enough how lucky I am to have discovered the way to health. I have lost over 15 inches and feel like a new woman. My joints are moving, I have a spring in my step and I know that if I continue to exercise for the rest of my like it will surely lead me back to the body I was meant to have and if I have to be a larger person then at least I will be a healthy one!!!"

Stehpanie E.

"I am 51 years old and in the throes of menopause. My husband is retired, recovering from heart bypass and gall bladder surgery. My job is extremely stressful and I have to drive into downtown Los Angeles every day. I need aerobics to keep me sane."

Lucy Y,

"I am 37 years old and feeling great! I started to exercise again about 3 months ago. Before that I had found every excuse why I couldn't get on a regular exercise program. And the longer I waited the more tired and heavier I got. It is true I do have a very busy schedule and it isn't always easy to get to the class on time, however, after getting back into my program I feel so much better. I have more energy, I'm more flexible, have better coordination and my self-esteem and confidence has gotten better. Sometimes I really have to make an effort to getting to class but believe me, it is worth it!!!"

Annette F.

"I am very committed to a regular exercise program for many reasons. It has been very helpful to me as a stress reduction method, particularly over the past few years. It also helps somewhat with weight control and muscle toning.

When I became a non-smoker about a year ago, it was very easy for me to gain weight because of the metabolic changes in my body. Actually, I usually didn't even have to eat the food - I could just look at it and I would gain weight - or so it seemed. I found that with a regular and more intensive exercise program, my weight became less of an issue.

Finally, and maybe most importantly, a regular exercise program seems to be linked to my feelings of well-being and self-esteem. I have had many trials and tribulations during my lifetime and have overcome several adversities. I heard once that life is like an onion - you peel it off one layer at a time. The analogy for me is that you can only work on one thing in your life at a time and basic needs come first. There was a time in my life when exercise was just not as important to me as some of the other issues in my life at that time. But time passes, we learn and mature. Exercise has become one of the latest steps for me in my continual growth process. I enjoy it a lot, feel healthy when I get a good work out and sweat a lot. I think that it will always remain an integral part of my life. Michele is good at keeping the momentum going and giving encouragement - and positive feedback is important."

Connie L.

"Aerobics is now part of my life. Without doing aerobics three times a week I feel lifeless and without energy to do the things that I enjoy. I highly recommend it to my friends and family."

Grace A.

"I did not start exercising until 2 years ago at the age of 42. Prior to that, I was basically sedentary. I had no energy, was easily tired which made me frequently depressed. I had pains in my joints, I was ready to retire. Since I started exercising, I've increased my energy level 100%. I feel so much stronger. My outlook in life is so much brighter, basically due to the fact that I have the energy to do things which were so difficult to do before. The physical benefits of exercise are obvious but I appreciate the benefits on my emotional state much more. I like myself better. The amount of time I invest in exercising is very minimal compared to the emotional benefits it provides me."

Margo P.

"Water exercise is great on building up my strength for soccer. It's also better for rehabilitating my muscles than weightlifting. I think it's more fun than weightlifting too. We have tons of fun!"

Karen M.

"I am an overweight housewife and mother of four young children. I started exercising to lose weight. I have continued for other reasons. Stress reduction, increased strength, stamina and a caring, well informed instructor have kept me going to classes."

Denise H.

"My friend invited me to come as her guest to her aerobics class. I accepted the invitation and the rest is history. I've been in a regular exercise program for over a year and have enjoyed the improved health benefits. I never thought I needed a regular exercise program since I was so young, at my ideal weight and had no health problems. I was wrong. Not only has my endurance improved but so has my self-image."

Bonnie C.

"I like and want to do fun things, especially outdoor activities that are physically demanding. Having children has enriched my life but has made it difficult to maintain my previous level of fitness. I have finally found that regularly scheduled exercise classes have filled a gap that helps me retain at least a basic level of fitness. Now I can participate in all the fun things I've always enjoyed doing with an emphasis on fun and less on work and pain."

Chris. B

"I think water exercise is great! You can work really hard and still laugh a lot between groans! It's also much easier on this 70 year old body."

Joyce G.

"Exercise for me doesn't always mean classroom aerobics. Variety is what keeps me exercising regularly. The structured classes keep my honest and committed to my goal of good health and fitness. Less structured walking and swimming exercise I use as 'fillers' because they can be done so easily and at most anytime and place.

I make it a habit to exercise daily by avoiding the use of elevators, escalators, people movers, taxi's, etc. I choose the stairs most often if they are safe, I park my car in a distant space rather than close up. When traveling I walk rapidly through the airports and I do my sightseeing on foot walking and enjoying the sights, sounds and smells of an unfamiliar place. I try to make exercise fun by incorporating it into my daily life in small doses and focusing on my ultimate goal of "quality of life".

I choose to exercise because I enjoy it's life enriching benefits; increased energy, self-confidence & self-esteem, physical ability, flexibility, stamina, agility, pride, reduced stress and tensions, etc., etc.,. etc. How can one not enjoy their 'quality of life' time when it produces such positive results?!"

Marty A.

"I like water aerobics because I enjoy it. I feel it has helped me tone up after losing all my weight. I also like the instructor. I feel tired but good after class."

Roberta B.

"I accredit aerobic exercise classes for contributing to my victories in tennis. I am 42 years old and play #1 singles on my 4.5 USTA Tennis Team. We went to the Sectionals and I won all my matches in straight sets. I felt no fatigue and I was very quick footed. Exercise has kept my weight down and kept me mentally alert.

I feel I can outlast my opponent in endurance alone and this is what gives me the edge. Now we are on our way to the Nationals representing Southern California!"

Janet G.

"I enjoy water aerobics. It has given me a whole new look at exercising. I feel so much better now that I am moving!"

Diana V.

"I exercise each day to feel good. I try to do some activity at least three or four times a week, or more. Eating right and exercising are all part of living a good sensible life. If you feel good, live good and smile each day, there is only room in your heart to love your fellow man and share the goodness of feeling good."

Jane F.

"I realized I should start working out when I had to unsnap the top button on my Levi's and when I was not able to tuck my shirt in my pants!"

Gilda R.

"I'm Sandy - I won't ever see the late parties again. Although I have a physical job, I found myself 45 lbs. overweight. After deciding to do something about losing the weight, I joined the aerobics class at my work. Working out has given me a feeling of accomplishment, more energy, added strength and I feel healthier. After 6 months I'm just 20 lbs. overweight and I go through my day with a more confident attitude. Now when I work out I feel it's a reward, not a job."

Sandy M.

"Have you ever felt tired, unattractive or simply less than together? Well, that's exactly what I feel like when my body is neglected. I have always enjoyed the benefits of exercising, such as energy, a good body, feeling on top of things. My problem is activating my physique when I'm dormant.

The story is always the same - with the little bit of asthma that I have; pushing myself beyond, for the first couple weeks is a must for me. I do enjoy testing my limits - I try to be smart about it. My asthma seems to adjust as my body gets into shape. Although there are days (i.e., smoggy) that I use my inhalator.

I've gone from being a consistent swimmer and a jogger to nothing for over 2 years. And then after having my first baby I hit bottom. I had had it with not feeling good about myself and my body. Since I've been exercising I've started feeling better and caring about myself again. Even my husband has noticed and doesn't mind caring for our 6 month old while I enjoy an hour of aerobics. I feel attractive and full of life, my honey can only love me more."

Chris B.

"The main reason I exercise is because I love to eat and hate to be fat. However, almost equally important is the way it makes me feel about myself. Exercise does wonders for my self-esteem, my posture, my energy levels, my ability to cope with both physical and mental stress, and my emotional stability. If it was a drug it would be illegal. Yet it's available to everyone and in such glorious variety. Although I have gone through periods of exercising on my own, I think it's more fun to exercise (at least some of the time) with other people; the trick is to keep looking until you find a compatible group. For me that means an aerobics class that's not a dance class in disguise (I really identified with that Reebok commercial: "This ain't no dance class"). I've also found that it's important to have a kind of exercise that I can do to get started again, for those times (holidays, vacation, illness) during which I've stopped or become irregular about

my primary exercise. Knowing that I can take a brisk walk for exercise is a great motivation for those times I'm feeling out of shape and dreading the idea of starting all over again. It surprised me to discover that having a gentle exercise like walking to fall back on makes it easier to keep exercise a regular part of my life, I think it stops me from panicking about lapses. One last thing, I really love having muscles."

Lisa D.

"My reasons for exercising are threefold. The main reason is HEALTH. When I exercise I work various parts of my body that I would not normally use, thus helping my heart, limbs, muscles and brain function better as a result. Another reason is to relieve stress. My job is very stressful and when I feel the tension mounting, I go and work it off. It's a marvelous stress reliever. Overall, I exercise to feel and look good. I never overdo it and the results are fantastic. Everyone should exercise."

Janice H.

"There are many reasons why I exercise. Years ago, the men used to walk by me and say, "What's up slim?". Now they walk by me and say, "What's up?".

Now at the age of 29 (soon to be 30) and over 200 lbs., I mainly exercise to tone and to lose weight. I enjoy exercising because my job is very stressful and I love to eat. Exercising helps me to release stress and feel relaxed. I recommend it to anyone that likes to feel good!!!"

Tammy B.

"The reasons I exercise are numerous. First and foremost, I would like to think I do it for my health. But I think it's vanity that's my biggest motivator. Nothing

makes my day like being able to go to a store and put on clothes that fit well and look good (jokingly). On the serious side, the health benefits I receive are well worth the effort and time that I put in. There's nothing more uplifting than knowing you can walk or run a few miles without feeling you're going to pass out. The overall feeling of wellness is a boost to my mental state. I've been an avid exerciser all of my life except for a few years during my early thirties and the quality of my life deteriorated seriously to a point where it was in danger. The main thing that pulled me through the brink was exercising regularly."

June B.

"...Let me tell you a little history of myself. I never had a weight problem, always weighed 99 lbs. up til age of 22, then had children. Highest weight then was 105 lbs. I always ate anything and everything I felt like eating. I wanted some meat on my body, couldn't get meat on my body. Then when I hit my middle 30's I started gaining weight but in the wrong places. I went up to 124 lbs. I was taking medication which I now know contributed to weight gain, plus I was never into fitness and never was watching what I should and should not eat. Well I joined a fitness program at work, used the stair master only, and didn't see any weight loss. then I decided to try aerobic classes. I lost 12 lbs. and feel great!!!

I have also encouraged my children to exercise as much as they can and the whole family eats more nutritious. Exercising makes me feel good about myself. I know I am doing something good for my body instead of abusing it. I might not have a body like the instructors' but I feel good about me."

Gloria M.

Maybe you can relate to some of these wonderful people. Each one was once where you are now. As you've already read, those who exercise regularly can list numerous benefits—and you can realize those benefits too. These benefits are enjoyed by a select group of regular exercisers, and you're on your way to becoming a member of that group as well!

CHAPTER REFLECTION

Date: _____

What did I learn from this chapter?

What will I do differently or apply this week?

How do I feel after completing this chapter?

YOUR PATH TO LASTING CHANGE

REFLECTION ACTIVITIES

Congratulations! You made it. Give yourself time to reflect upon your overall journey here. Write down answers to the following questions:

What were my biggest breakthroughs during this process?

What habits have I built that I want to maintain?

What thoughts or beliefs helped or hurt me?

How has my view of fitness or health changed?

What am I grateful for in this process?

What is my intention for tomorrow, next week, in future months?

What did I learn about myself through this whole process?

STAGES OF CHANGE

Revisit the Stages of Change model you saw in Chapter 1. What stage do you see yourself at now? Did you move forward, back or stay the same? Why do you think that is?

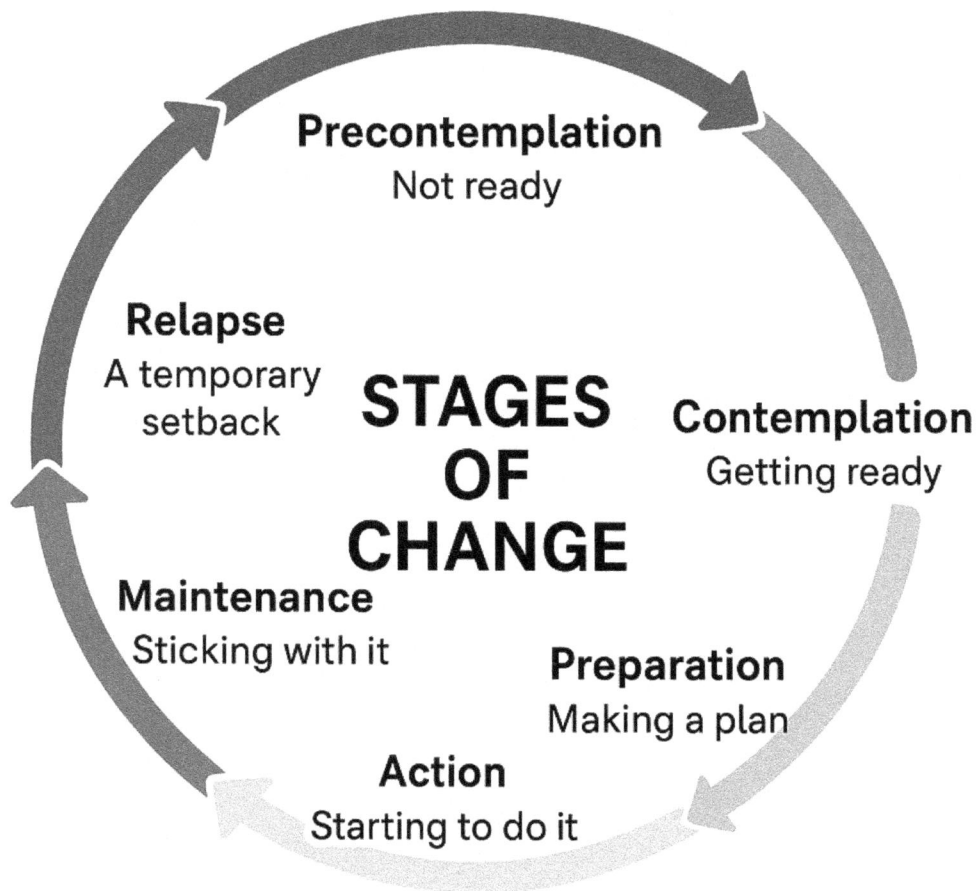

Precontemplation
Not ready

Contemplation
Getting ready

Relapse
A temporary setback

STAGES OF CHANGE

Maintenance
Sticking with it

Preparation
Making a plan

Action
Starting to do it

FITNESS DIARY

Now that you have completed the entire workbook, use the following pages to begin recording a simple, daily fitness diary. Write down whether you exercised each day, what type of exercise you did and how you felt about it. Track your progress over time to see if you are holding steady or slipping backward. Catching a lack of motivation or an interruption in your program early can help keep you exercising long term. Once you run out of space here, continue in your own journal.

Date: _____

Thoughts/Feelings_____

_____

_____

_____

Date: _____

Thoughts/Feelings_____

_____

_____

_____

Date: _____

Thoughts/Feelings_____

_____

_____

_____

Date: _____

Thoughts/Feelings_____

_____

_____

_____

Date: _____

Thoughts/Feelings_____

_____

_____

_____

Date: _____

Thoughts/Feelings_____

_____

_____

_____

Date: _____

Thoughts/Feelings_____

_____

_____

_____

Date: _____

Thoughts/Feelings_____

_____

_____

_____

Date: _____

Thoughts/Feelings_____

_____

_____

_____

Date: _____

Thoughts/Feelings_____

_____

_____

_____

Date: _____

Thoughts/Feelings_____

_____

_____

_____

Date: _____

Thoughts/Feelings_____

_____

_____

_____

Date: _____

Thoughts/Feelings_____

_____

_____

_____

Date: _____

Thoughts/Feelings_____

_____

_____

_____

Date: _____

Thoughts/Feelings_____

_____

_____

_____

Date: _____

Thoughts/Feelings_____

_____

_____

_____

Date: _____

Thoughts/Feelings_____

_____

_____

_____

Date: _____

Thoughts/Feelings_____

_____

_____

_____

Date: _____

Thoughts/Feelings_____

_____

_____

_____

Date: _____

Thoughts/Feelings_____

_____

_____

_____

Date: _____

Thoughts/Feelings_____

_____

_____

_____

Date: _____

Thoughts/Feelings_____

_____

_____

_____

Date: _____

Thoughts/Feelings_____

_____

_____

_____

APPENDIX 1

Contraindicated Exercises

Familiarize yourself with stretches and exercises that are dangerous and outdated. Especially if you are just starting an exercise program. These are still used by those who have not kept up to date on safety.

Stretches:

1. <u>Full Neck Circles</u> - Stressful on the cervical vertebrae. Eliminate backward portion of the circle, rolling just to the sides and front, to prevent damage.

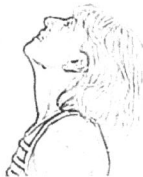 NO
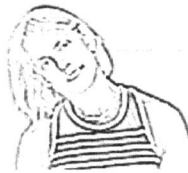 YES

2. <u>Straight Leg Toe Touches</u> - Although popular, reaching over and touching the toes is not the preferred way to stretch the hamstrings. In individuals with tight back muscles, the stretch is being directed into the lower back, not legs. Hanging over with hands unsupported means the person lacks flexibility and thus needs to stretch the hamstring muscles, not strain ligaments of the lower back. Modify by doing the stretch on the floor/chair, bending knees, or reaching over one leg alone.

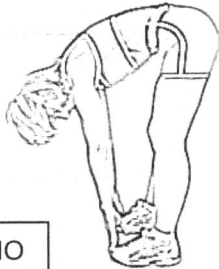 NO
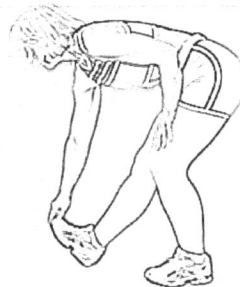 YES

3. Knee Sitting - Hyperflexion of the knee joint is not the safest way to stretch the quadricep muscles. There are various ways to stretch the quadriceps without compressing the knee joints under the full weight of the body.

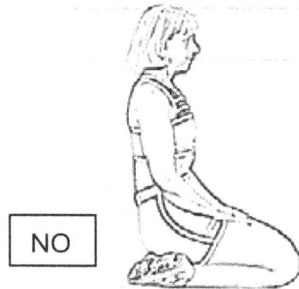

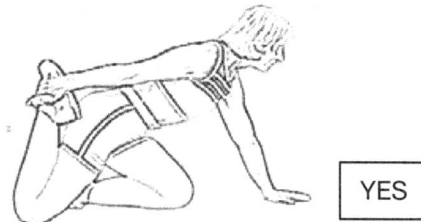

NO

YES

4. Back Hyperextension - Back bends and extreme hyperextension can put stress on vertebrae. A safer alternative is to support the back during extension or lift the back from a face down position.

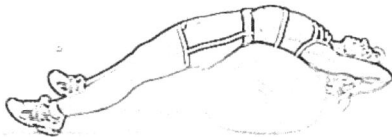

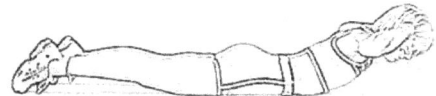

5. Hurdler's Stretch - One leg is stretched straight out in front while the other knee is bent with the foot facing backwards. Leads to joint instability by overstretching the medial ligament of the back leg. Correct by just changing the position of the back leg so foot is facing straight leg instead of pointing backwards.

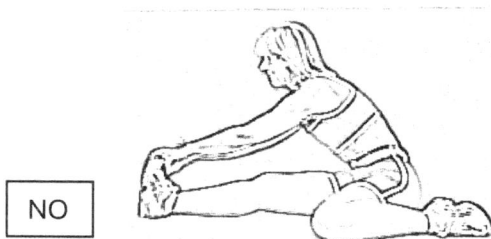

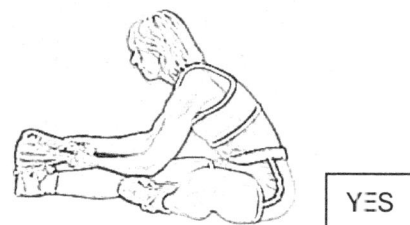

NO

YES

6. <u>Forward Flexion with Trunk Rotation</u> - "Windmills" are dangerous for the lower back and knees. Rotation places pressure on discs in the back. Safer alternatives include placing the hands on the knees and turning the upper body to one side and then the other.

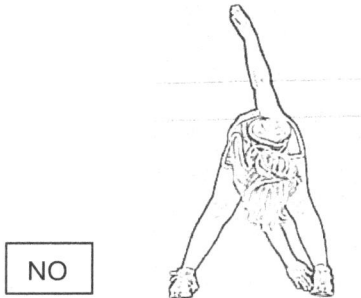

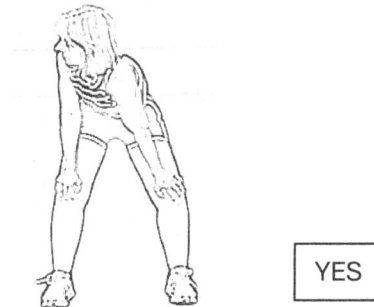

NO   YES

Strength Exercises:

<u>Straight Leg Sit Ups</u> - Strain is put on iliopsoas muscle (the crease of the hip) which can lead to an abnormal lumbar curve and back pain. Always bend knees while doing any kind of abdominal crunch.

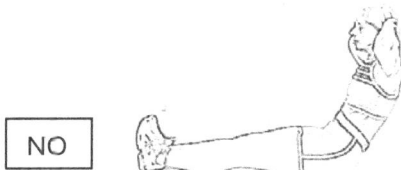

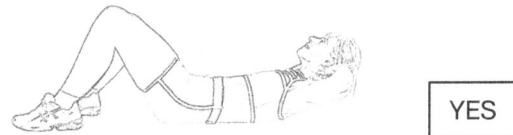

NO   YES

<u>Deep Knee bends/Full squats</u> - Produces stress on knee joint and ligaments - which over time can weaken the knee. Keep the angle of the knee at 90 degrees or less. Weight of the hips should be kept over the heels.

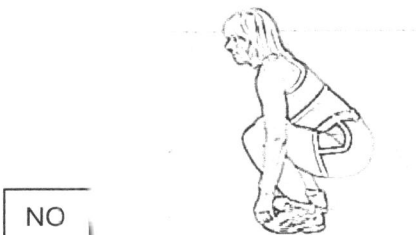

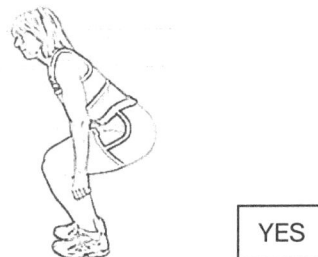

NO   YES

As a general rule DO NOT:

- Lock or compress joints
- Bounce while stretching
- Swing or use jerky movements, especially with any kind of weighted item
- Arch back excessively or extend neck backwards

APPENDIX 2
Strength Routines

Always warm up gently before doing any of these exercises. Nothing strenuous — just move around for a few minutes to get your blood circulating so your muscles are warm and ready to work.

These strengthening exercises are very basic and can be done either standing or sitting in a chair. If you don't have arm weights, use small soup cans until you build up strength — or nothing at all until you feel ready. Building and maintaining strength is essential for staying independent throughout life. You want to be able to sit down and stand up easily and get up from the floor without needing help. Staying strong means staying self-reliant—and out of nursing homes.

As you exercise, focus on keeping your body tight and your posture tall. The photo on the left shows the starting position; the photo on the right shows the movement. Repeat each exercise at least 12 times, working up to 24. If you're only doing one side of the body, be sure to repeat the exercise on the other side. When an exercise becomes too easy, add a bit of weight or increase your repetitions.

Strength Plan #1

STANDING/HOLDING CHAIR

Shoulders – Upright Rows

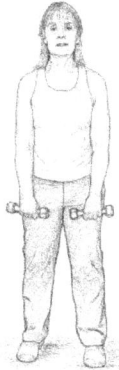

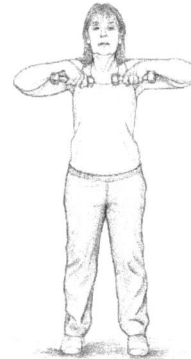

Stand with knees bent, palms facing down

Slowly raise both arms until hands are underneath chin and elbows point wide open, then return to start position

Biceps – Curls

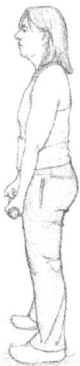

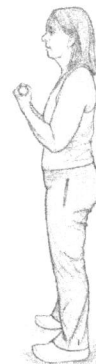

Stand with knees bent, palms face up

Slowly raise one or both arms until hands are close to chest, then lower them

Triceps – Kickbacks

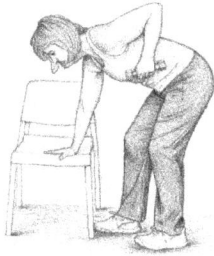

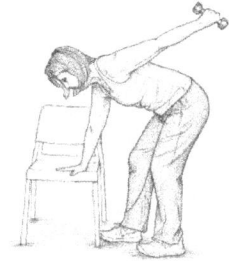

Hold chair and lift other elbow up,
keeping arm against body

Extend arm all the way back
and return to start position

Back – One Arm Rows

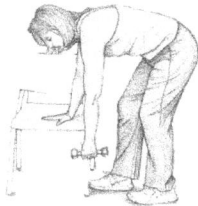

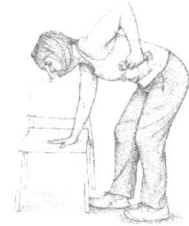

Support yourself with one arm on
a chair, let other arm hang

Pull the weight up toward
your waist then slowly lower it

Chest – Front Squeeze

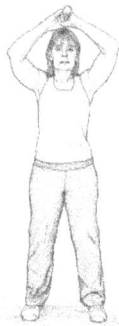

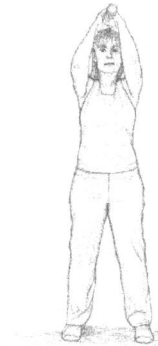

Stand with knees bent, weight
overhead and elbows wide
apart

Squeeze the elbows towards
each other while keeping the
weight overhead

Legs – Squats

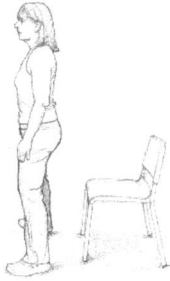

Stand with feet wide apart, toes pointing open or straight ahead

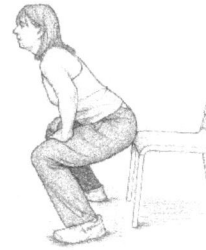

→

Lower into a sitting position as far as you comfortably can then rise again

Legs – Lunges

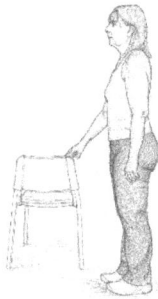

Stand with feet together. Hold on to a chair or wall if needed

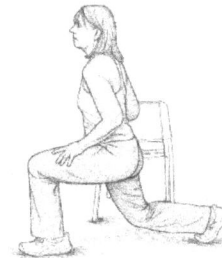

→

Step as far forward as you can and drop other knee towards the ground. Return to start, then repeat other leg.

Calf – Raises

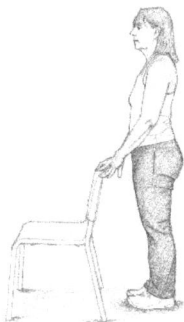

Stand with knees bent, holding on to a chair or wall

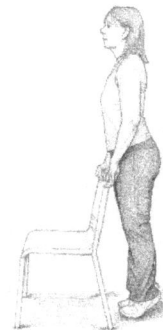

→

Lift both heels off the ground as far as you can, then return to start position

Abductors – Side Leg Lifts

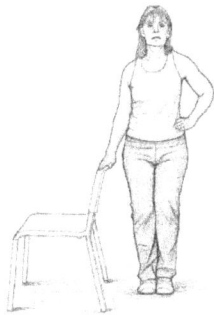

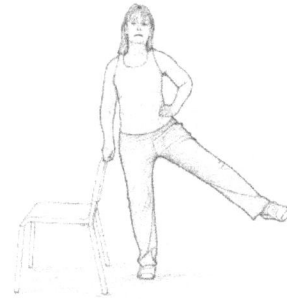

Hold on to a chair or wall with
both knees slightly bent

Lift the outside leg to the side
then back down. Do not go so
high that you tip to the side

Obliques – Side Bend

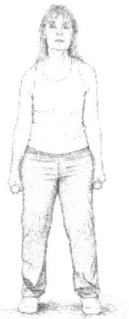

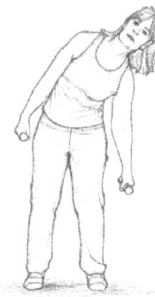

Stand with feet slightly apart
with weight in one hand

Keep knees bent, lean over to
the side and then stand back
up. Keep arms relaxed.

Abdominals – Seated Crunch

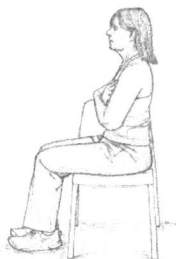

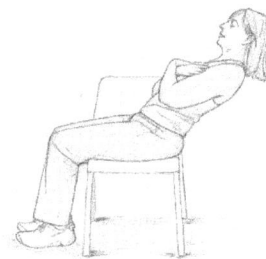

Sit sideways on a chair with arms
crossed over chest

Keep feet on floor and lean
back as far as you can, then
sit up

Strength Plan #2

SITTING/FLOOR

Shoulders – Bent Arm Lateral Raises

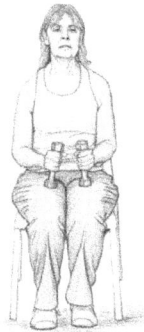

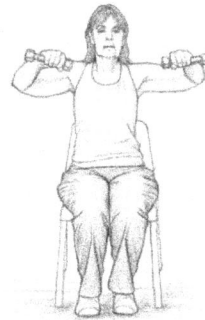

Stand or sit in a chair with a weight in each hand

→

With elbows bent, open arms outward to shoulder height, then lower

Biceps – Preacher Curl

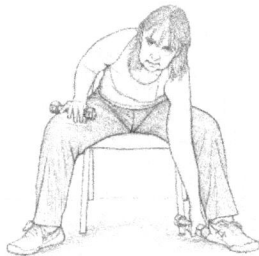

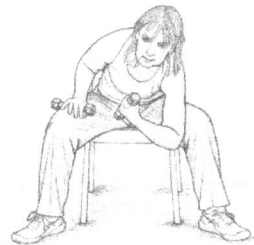

Sit with legs open, press back of upper arm against thigh

→

Curl weight toward opposite shoulder, then lower. Repeat other arm

Triceps – Overhead Extension

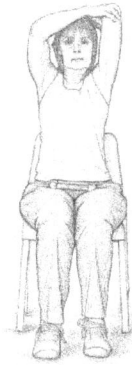

Sit with one arm holding a weight, let arm with weight bend behind head

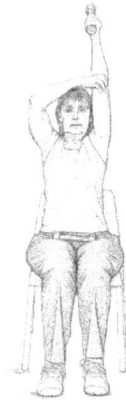

Brace arm with other hand then lift and lower from elbow

Upper Back – Rear Lateral Raise

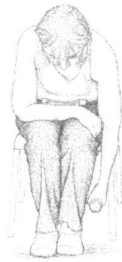

Sit and lean forward with weight hanging down to side

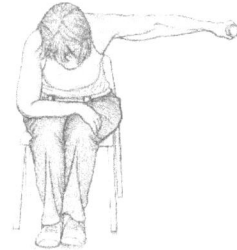

Keep elbow slightly bent then open arm out to side. Do not swing.

Back – Bird Dog

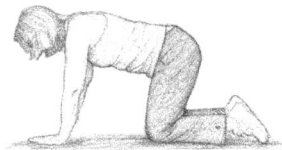

Start on hands and knees, keep back lifted

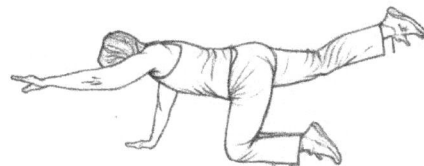

Extend opposite arm and leg. Bring back in. Repeat other side.

Pectorals – Flyes

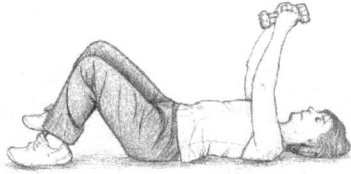

Lie on back with arms up, palms facing in. Keep elbows slightly bent

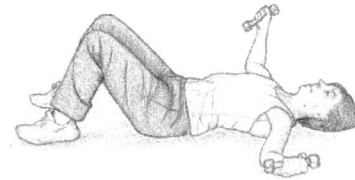

Bring both arms open, down until elbows hit floor, then lift

Glutes – Hip Lifts

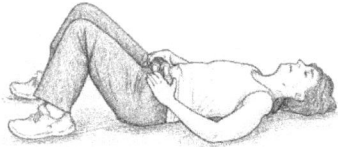

Lie on back with feet apart. Use weight on top of pelvis

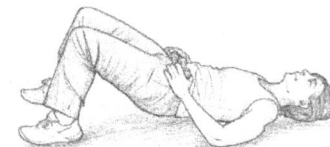

Lift hips up by pressing through feet, then lower to start position

Adductors – Leg V's

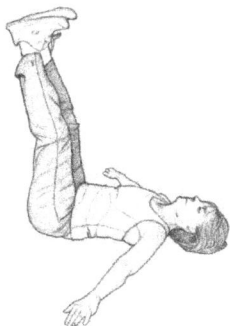

Lie on back with both legs in air, knees stay bent

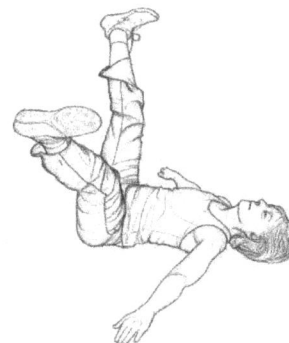

Toes point to face. Open legs as far as you can, then close

Quadriceps – Leg Extensions

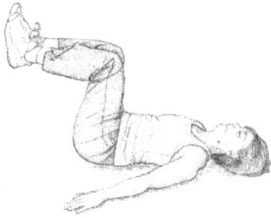

Lie on back with feet in air and
knees bent at a right angle

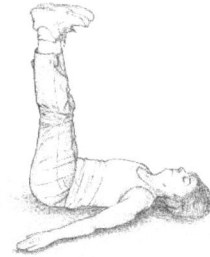

Lift both legs until straight,
then lower and repeat

Abdominals – Crunches

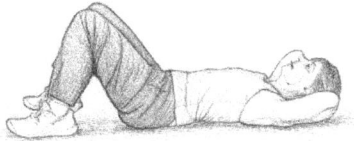

Lie on back with hands behind head,
elbows wide open, chin up

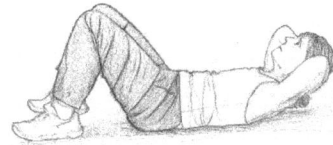

Lay head in your hands. Lift
shoulders off floor without
pulling on head.

Obliques – Diagonal Crunch

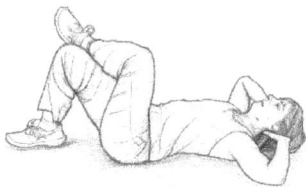

Lie on back with one foot on
opposite knee, elbows open

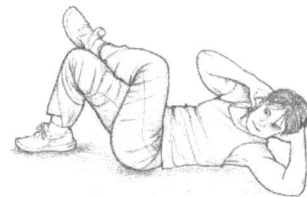

Lift diagonally reaching for top
knee, then return to floor

221

APPENDIX 3
Stretch Routines

Do your stretches at the end of your workout, not at the beginning. You want to be warm so your muscles, ligaments, and tendons can safely elongate without risk of injury. Remember, don't bounce when you stretch. Instead, hold the position at the point of mild tightness.

There are two sample plans: one standing, and one sitting or floor-based. Choose whichever feels most comfortable. You can alternate between them or substitute a stretch from the other plan if something doesn't feel right. For each stretch, hold where you feel the most tightness for 30–60 seconds, then switch sides.

Stretch Plan #1

STANDING/HOLDING CHAIR

Shoulder – Chest Squeeze

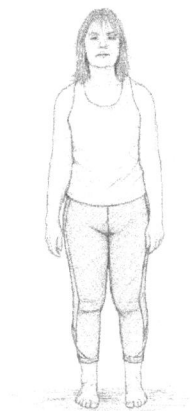

Stand in a relaxed position

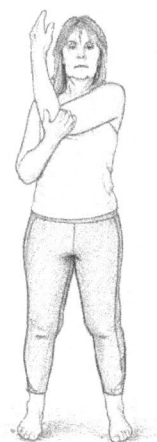

Hold elbow with opposite hand.
Raise arm and squeeze inward
across the chest

Biceps – Arm Rotation Stretch

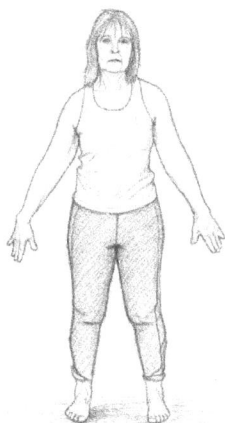

Stand with knees bent, palms face back

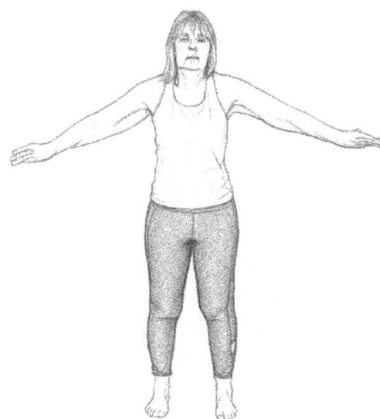

Raise both arms to the side, rotating
the entire arm so palms face up

Triceps – Overhead Stretch

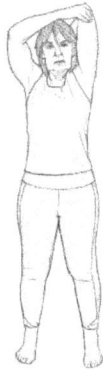

Put one hand behind the head
and grab elbow with the other

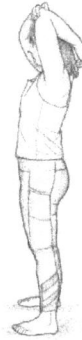

Press the arm backwards with
the front arm

Back – Forward Reach

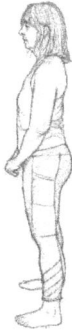

Stand with hands clasped and
knees bent

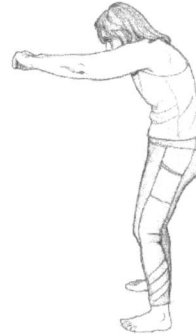

Round out your upper back
while pressing arms forward

Chest – Clasp Behind

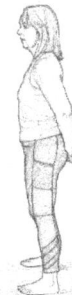

Hold hands together behind
your back

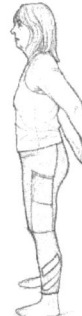

Pull both shoulders backwards
and lift arms away from body

Hamstring/Glutes – Sit-Backs

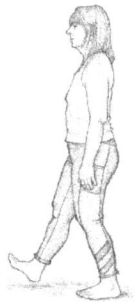

Stand and place one heel out in
front of your body

→

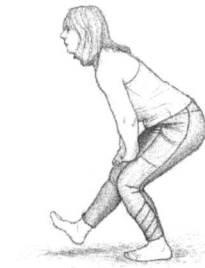

Keeping knees together, sit
back as low as you can go

Calf – Standing Calf Stretch

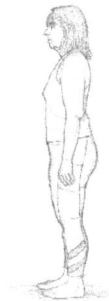

Stand with feet together. Hold
on to a chair or wall if needed

→

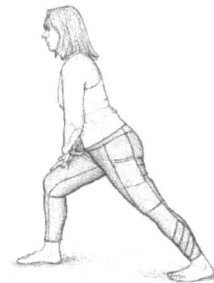

Step backwards as far as you
can. Keep toes forward, heel
flat

Quadriceps – Seated Lean Back

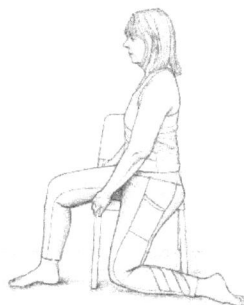

Sit sideways on a chair and let
one leg hang off the front

→

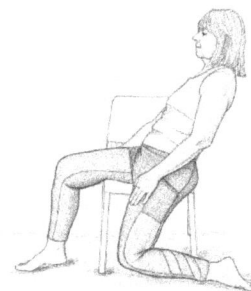

Holding the chair, lean upper
body back keeping leg still

Abductors – Seated Cross-Leg Stretch

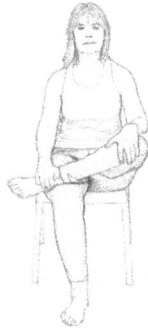

Sit upright, one foot on opposite thigh

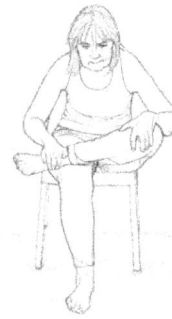

→

Lean forward and hold

Adductors – Press Outs

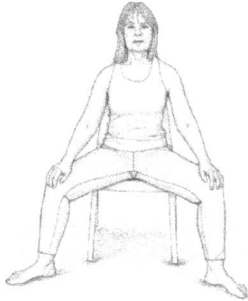

Sit upright with legs wide open

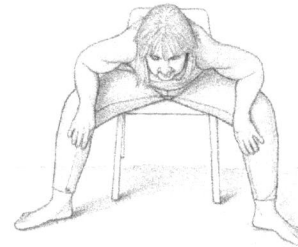

→

Lean forward while pressing both legs open with arms

Obliques – Single Arm Overhead Reach

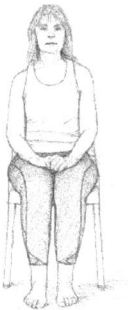

Sit or stand

→

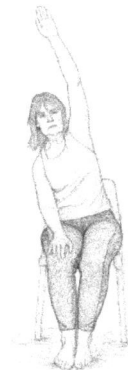

Reach one arm overhead as high as possible then lean to side, diagonally

Abdominals – Double Arm Overhead Reach

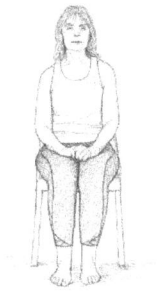

Sit or stand with hands clasped

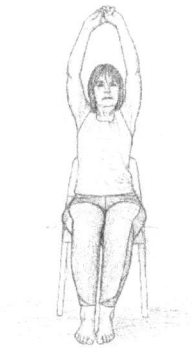

Reach both arms up
overhead as far as possible

Stretch Plan #2

SITTING/FLOOR

Trapezius – Neck Stretch

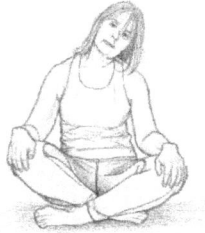

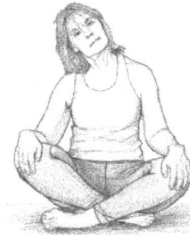

$\longrightarrow$

Sit upright. Tilt head toward one shoulder as far as comfortable, hold

Then tilt your head to the opposite shoulder and hold

Deltoid – Arm Across Chest

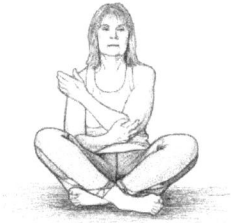

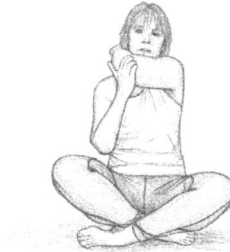

$\longrightarrow$

Hold one elbow across the body with the opposite hand

Use that hand to gently pull the arm up and in, around neck

Adductors - Butterfly

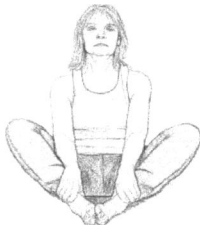

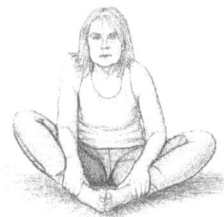

$\longrightarrow$

Sit tall, feet together. Back is straight, hold ankles

Press both knees open while leaning forward to floor. Keep back straight

Triceps – Elbow Press

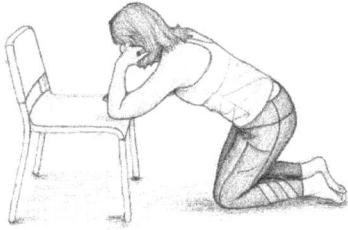

Place back of elbow on a chair, wall or floor

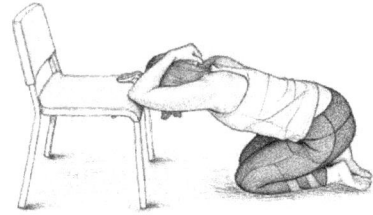

Sink gently into the stretch until your elbow moves slightly past your head

Biceps – Leaning Arm Rotation

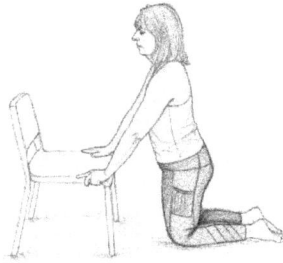

Using a chair or while kneeling on the floor, place hands shoulder-width apart, thumbs facing inward

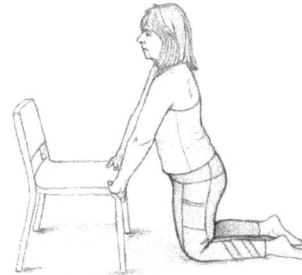

Rotate your arms so the thumbs turn outward, feeling the stretch through your arms

Lats – Round Ball

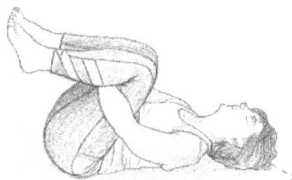

While on your back, place hands under both knees

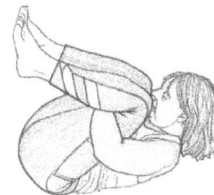

Lift shoulders and pull your legs in close, aiming for knees to move toward face

Pectorals/Obliques – Back Twist

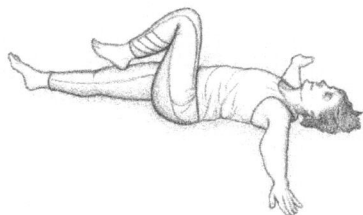

Lie on back with arms out to side and one knee lifted

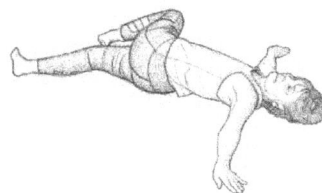

Drop the bent knee across your body while keeping both shoulders on the ground

Hamstrings – Leg Pull

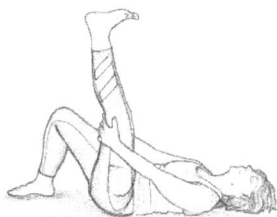

Lie on back with one leg in the air, hands clasped under it (or use a towel)

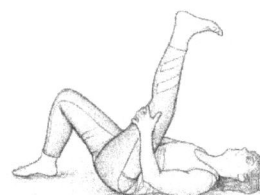

Pull leg towards face, keeping toes pulled in and leg as straight as possible

Abductors – Cross Leg Lift

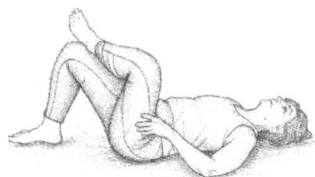

Lie on back with one foot on top of the other knee

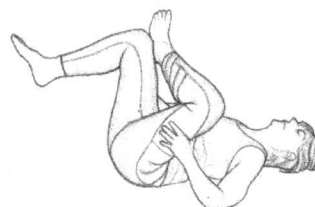

Lift both legs until you feel a stretch on the outside of the top leg

Quadriceps – Knee Turn

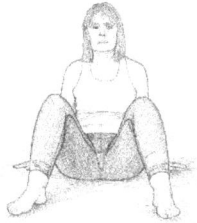

Sit with feet wide apart

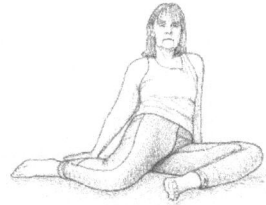

Tilt both legs to one side, pressing back knee down while lifting same side hip. Repeat other side

Abdominals – Straight Line Stretch

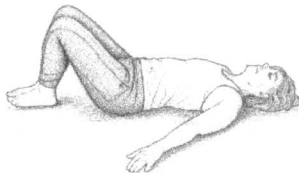

Lie on back

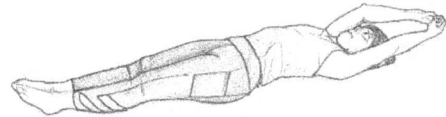

Reach arms and legs in opposite directions as far as you can

Obliques – Waist Stretch

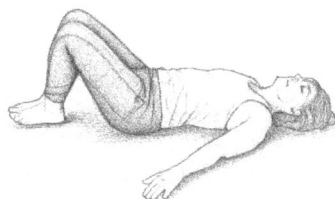

Lie on back with feet and knees together, arms open to side

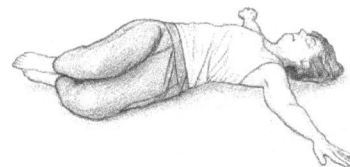

Tilt the hips to one side while keeping arms open. Repeat other side

ABOUT THE AUTHOR

Michele Silence, M.A., is a fitness professional, educator, and lifelong advocate for healthy living. She combines her master's in Clinical/Sport Psychology with over 40 years of experience helping people of all ages move, grow, and thrive.

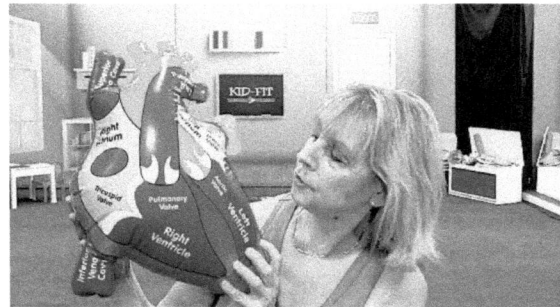

She is the founder of the KID-FIT Preschool Health and Fitness Organization and creator of KID-FIT, P.E. Classes for Preschoolers. Michele also directs the annual KID-FIT Family Fun Run 1K/5K in Southern California, inspiring children and families to embrace healthy lifestyle habits.

Michele teaches virtual adult fitness classes focused on strength, balance, flexibility, and functional movement. She has written for national fitness magazines, authored continuing education courses for educators, lectured at various conferences, and is a fitness news columnist.

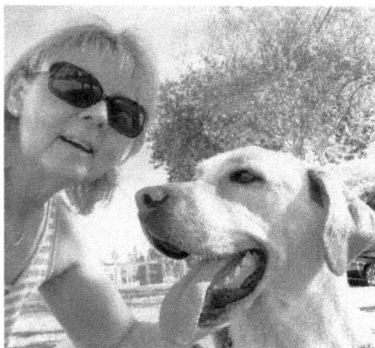

A long-time vegan, Michele promotes healthy, plant-based living and shares her home with her dogs and cats, who inspire her daily with their energy and joy.

Her programs are practical, supportive, and designed for real life, helping anyone overcome barriers and enjoy movement at any age.

For questions about this book or business inquiries, email michele@kid-fit.com